In the middle of cultural upheaval and institutional uncertainty, Marc's call to pivot comes as a voice crying in the wilderness. With remarkable clarity, he diagnoses the challenges arising for our culture and the church, exposing not only what is, but also illuminating what could and should be. More than an insightful analysis, this book is a clarion call to courageous action, offering readers both the vision and the tools needed to navigate change faithfully and effectively.

— Jor-El Godsey, President, Heartbeat International

Pivot enables the prolife movement to adapt to a new environment and a new battle after the fall of *Roe*. As a longtime prolife educator and strategist myself, I can tell you that this book will empower you. It is both realistic and principled. Marc doesn't waste a single word. You will learn something on every page, and you will come away convinced that there is always a way to win!

— Frank Pavone, National Director, Priests for Life; President, National Prolife Religious Council

In a world where abortion has been normalized as an acceptable part of the human experience, Dr. Marc Newman has written a field manual for the front lines. Drawing on the truth of 2 Corinthians 10:3–5, he equips readers to demolish strong-held arguments with wisdom, wit, irrefutable facts, and unwavering conviction. Dr. Newman isn't merely responding to the culture—he's helping lead the charge to reclaim the truth that will set us free and save lives.

— Nicku Bruce, Executive Director, Real Choices Women's Center, NV

Pivot is a masterful blueprint for the pro-life movement in a post-Roe world. It charts a real-world map for success between distractions that seek to derail efforts to save children, whether whole life advocates on the left or immediately on the right. Read this book if you want reality rather than fiction.

— Scott Klusendorf, President, Life Training Institute, author of *The Case for Life*

In *Pivot*, Newman nails it. He presents the very real problems the pro-life movement faces in a post-Dobbs world. However, he does so with clarity and hope by pointing to the pivots necessary for our movement to recapture momentum, change culture, and end the violence of abortion in our nation once and for all.

— Trevor Polo, Executive Director, Protect Life Michigan

Pivot is a wake-up call for pastors and churches tempted to coast after *Dobbs*. Marc Newman makes a compelling case that the fight over abortion didn't end—it just moved, migrating to pills and shield laws and telehealth, while too many of us looked away. Dr. Newman refuses to let the church off the hook for its silence. He insists that good intentions mean nothing without action. This book is a rallying cry for those of us who already believe life is sacred but who need to move from conviction to action. I've known Marc for years and this book is exactly what I'd expect from him: direct, deeply researched, and impossible to read passively. Pastors and church leaders, this one belongs on your shelf.

— Dan Spencer, President, Tennessee Baptist Conference (SBC); Senior Pastor, First Baptist Church of Sevierville, Tennessee

With *Pivot*, Marc Newman provides clarity to our Post-Roe reality, then proposes a positive (and more important) *doable* path to winning back our culture for life in *this* generation. If every life-affirming Christian reads this book and chooses "Yes" to just one of the practical action steps Marc outlines in *Pivot*, the results could be beyond anything we can imagine.

— Kirk Walden, author of *The Wall* and *Saving Samaria*.

I would love to put this book into the hands of every elected official who states they vote "pro-life," but when asked "why?" they have no answer. I want every person who has ever said to me, "what can I do to help?" to read this book. Marc clearly communicates the "why's", "how's "and "who's" of the Pro-life issue in such a way that everyone can be fully informed, equipped to respond and pivot from being a bystander to taking action in a meaningful way.

— Erin Rogers, Executive Director, Bakersfield Pregnancy Center, CA

This is war. After Dobbs, the abortion industry didn't retreat—it pivoted with chemical death pills, shield laws, firebombed centers, and brazen lies. I've battled it for decades. This book rips the mask off with hard evidence, raw stories, and unapologetic Scripture. *Pivot* delivers the hard-hitting strategies we need: truth-telling language, bold church action, enforceable laws, and boots-on-the-ground advances into hostile territory. The fight is now. Read it—and fight.

— Rev. Troy Newman, President, Operation Rescue; Founder, Center for Medical Progress

We all worked, prayed, and voted for the day Roe v. Wade would be overturned. While we celebrated on June 24, 2022, the culture of death pivoted to an even deadlier strategy. Marc Newman describes its strategy and methods. But more importantly, Marc lays out the pivot that advocates for life must take to win elections, take back the culture, value women, and save precious preborn babies.

— Melissa Clement, Executive Director, Nevada Right to Life

Pivot is an exceptional resource for anyone who wants to understand the abortion debate beyond slogans and headlines. Marc Newman presents a thoughtful, well-researched examination of abortion, the legal landscape surrounding it, and the ethical questions at its core. Rather than relying on emotional appeals, *Pivot* encourages readers to examine evidence, history, and reasoned arguments. I proudly and highly recommend it.

— Victoria Robinson, CEO, Reassemble; author of *They Lied to Us*

Pivot provides thoughtful, well-researched insight into the abortion issue while challenging readers to consider how each of us can play a meaningful role in creating change. It doesn't just inform; it inspires action. This is a must-read for anyone who desires to help build a culture that values and protects life. If we truly want to make a difference and stand for the dignity of every innocent human being, this book is an important place to start.

— Valerie Millsapps, CEO, Pregnancy Resource Center, TN, author of *A Voice That Kills*

Marc Newman, in *Pivot*, not only identifies the major battlefronts facing the pro-life movement but also offers practical, actionable solutions. He does so with a motivating message that strengthens the resolve of those already fighting the battle for life while encouraging those on the sidelines to step in and get involved.

— Amber Singleton, Executive Director, Arkansas Right to Life

Wow - the pro-life community needs this wisdom and insightful look at this time. We have shifted, pivoted, and changed everything possible, but we need the church, legislators, and friends to pivot with us. The myths, the lies and rogue groups have tried to control the narrative and we need sanity. Marc is that sanity. It so encouraged me to read this roadmap of where we have been and where we need to go.... together. The attacks continue, but now we see attacks from places we never imagined. We need to approach education differently, we need to approach legislation differently, we need embrace the counsel in this book as the way forward. If you haven't read anything in a while about what is happening in the Prolife world, this is the book.

— Jana Pinson, Executive Director, Pregnancy Center of the Coastal Bend, TX

Pivot challenges us to examine not only the culture around us, but also ourselves. It reveals how, even as pro-life advocates, we have often accepted, aligned with, and adopted the deceptive language and narratives of the abortion movement without realizing it. This book is a fresh and compelling call to rethink how we engage one of the most important human rights issues of our time. Through thoughtful research, practical tools, and a compassionate yet unwavering commitment to truth, this book equips readers to become more effective advocates for life.

— Connie W. Coleman, Consultant, Coach, Christian Communicator

PIVOT

PIVOT

FIVE STRATEGIC SHIFTS TO WIN THE STATE-BY-STATE BATTLE FOR LIFE

MARC NEWMAN

AUTHOR OF *CONTENDERS*

Refocus PRESS

Sevierville, Tennessee

Pivot

Published by Refocus Press, Sevierville, TN 37862.

For bulk purchases, contact Refocus Press at https://refocuspress.com

Cover Desiga: Daniel O. Ojedokun
Book Design: Irena Kalcheva

Printed in the United States of America

ISBN: 978-1-7351962-4-4 (paperback)
ISBN: 978-1-7351962-5-1 (hardcover)
ISBN: 978-1-7351962-6-8 (ebook)

To Bob Foust,
whose endless encouragement
and tireless efforts on behalf of preborn children
are a source of motivation to all fortunate enough to know him

Contents

Acknowledgments

There are no three people in pro-life work whom I bounce more ideas off of than Scott Klusendorf, president of Life Training Institute; John Ensor, president of PassionLife; and Kirk Walden, national pro-life speaker and writer. All three provide me with an endless source of encouragement and are full of good humor, both important character traits in this line of work. I am grateful for their friendship.

Jor-El Godsey, president of Heartbeat International, provided excellent feedback on *Pivot*, just as he did on *Contenders*. He is a cheerful, effective warrior for life.

Cindy Viscardis, my Outreach Coordinator, keeps the schedule organized, pleasantly (though sometimes doggedly) interacts with event sponsors, and generally runs most of the day-to-day at Speaker for Life. I wouldn't have had time to write this book without her efforts.

Huge thanks to Jana Chapman, who pesters me for my calendar so she can coordinate with more than a hundred intercessors at our church who regularly pray for my events. I never asked her to do this; she just recognized the need and did it. You don't know how much that means to me.

To Gloria Leyda, my agent at Ambassador Speakers Bureau, thank you for continuing with me for many years and connecting me to so many great speakers and leaders.

As always, thanks to Grace Denny and Arthur Ellison. If not for you, I never would have entered this life-saving, life-affirming work. It changed my life.

Thanks to Steve Halliday, my editor, for his expertise in molding this book into its final form. I can't imagine publishing a book without him.

And to my other editor and proofreader, my beautiful wife, Sharon, who pored over this book more than once and saved me from a number of potentially embarrassing mistakes. Any that remain are entirely my fault. Your patience, love, and care for me are beyond measure. None of the work I do would be possible without you.

Thank you to all of the executive directors, CEOs, staff, and volunteers at all of the pregnancy help centers and clinics I have been privileged to work alongside over the years. Some of you are mentioned in the following pages, but all of you represent the kind of tireless, optimistic warriors this book is designed to produce.

Finally, all praise, honor, and glory to Almighty God, the true Giver of Life.

INTRODUCTION

What This Book Isn't, What It Is, and What to Expect in the End

For nearly forty years, I taught rhetoric, argumentation and debate, and public speaking at the college and university level. Alongside teaching, I also worked alongside pregnancy help centers and clinics and national and regional pro-life organizations, training their executive directors and staff to speak on behalf of their voiceless clients: children who reside in the wombs of their mothers. I continue to keynote fundraising banquets, train pastors, and teach pro-life apologetics.

In 2020 I wrote *Contenders: A Church-wide Strategy to Unmask Abortion, Defeat Its Advocates, Empower Christians, and Change the World*, aimed squarely at pro-life messengers. It offers a detailed, step-by-step approach to dismantling the claims of abortion advocates. It also contains a clear guide to crafting presentations, something I believe was missing in many other books on pro-life advocacy. Most books dealing with pro-life apologetics presented argument after argument but spent very little time explaining how to craft presentations designed to present all that material effectively. In *Contenders* I wanted to fill that gap.

After publishing *Contenders*, I didn't know whether I would ever write another book dealing with abortion. I believed I'd done a good job, the lines of argument are clear, and several other excellent pro-life apologetics books exist, especially the second edition of *The Case for Life*, written by my friend and colleague, Scott Klusendorf. The time was right, I thought, to finish a novel I'd been working on for years, or maybe write a rhetorical analysis of Christmas movies (as a trained rhetorical critic who loves Christmas, it seemed like a perfect fit).

But then the *Dobbs* decision came down, accomplishing what many people believed would never happen: it overturned *Roe v. Wade*. Suddenly, a dramatic shift took place in the landscape of the abortion battle.

I put my other writing projects on hold.

What Happened?

Roe v. Wade had made it nearly impossible for states to pass any meaningful protections for children in the womb, anywhere in the country. But after *Roe's* reversal, what had been a single, monolithic national policy immediately fractured into fifty pieces. *Dobbs* freed all states to make their own determinations regarding abortion. Rather than creating a static mosaic of pro-life and pro-abortion states, *Dobbs* introduced an ongoing, dynamic power struggle over abortion.

Pro-life forces had been so laser-focused on overturning *Roe* that, once it happened, many didn't know what to do next. Abortion advocates, taking their cue from Ruth Bader Ginsburg, who always held that *Roe* was poorly reasoned, had been planning. (The leak of the *Dobbs* decision months before its publication also gave pro-aborts advanced preparation time.)[1] Books such as Robin Marty's *Handbook for a Post-Roe America* (now in its second edition) laid the groundwork not only for securing abortion in pro-abortion states, but also how to take the fight over abortion into pro-life states.

Watching abortion advocates making headway and seeing pro-life advocates often fighting last decade's battles constrained me to dive back into the research. *Pivot* is my response. Because you elected to purchase and read this book, I want to be clear about what this book is not, what it is, and some of my expectations for those who read it.

What This Book Is Not

I wish you could see my office. Actually, I'm glad you can't. Even on the best of days, it has that "absent-minded professor" look; but as I put the finishing touches on *Pivot*, it looks like a research graveyard.

Observing my office, I see many books and hundreds of articles that I read and marked up. While I intended to use them all, they simply would not fit into a book that had a marketable page count. As the days approached to submit this manuscript, new articles kept popping into view. I had to recall a piece of sage advice offered by an academic colleague: "At some point the research must stop and the writing begins."

Not Exhaustive

Pivot is not exhaustive. It represents strategies and tactics carefully selected as actions that will make a substantial difference. I could have addressed other side issues, but at some point, authors must give up on being exhaustive to avoid exhausting their readers. All the greatest ideas on paper will make no difference if people don't read them. If *Pivot* whets your appetite to tackle this issue more thoroughly, other articles and books can move you further down the trail. Trust me, this book contains enough ideas and actions to keep you engaged for quite a while.

Not 'Just Another Apologetics Book'

While this book contains many arguments, it is not primarily a book of pro-life apologetics. I already wrote that book (or at least, a substantial portion of *Contenders* focuses on apologetics). One entire section in my previous book discusses how abortion advocates argue and how pro-life advocates can respond with evidence and analysis. *Contenders* covers the humanity and personhood of preborn children, discusses hard cases (such as rape and incest), shows the impacts of pregnancy and how they are used as a rationale for abortion, describes the policy implications of abortion, and then unmasks the extremism of abortion advocates.

I heartily recommend many other great pro-life apologetics books. Randy Alcorn's *Pro-Life Answers to Pro-Choice Arguments* is a classic. If you like Socratic dialogues, or just a good read, Peter Kreeft's *The Unaborted Socrates* fills the bill. Christopher Kaczor's excellent book, *The Ethics of Abortion*, is in its third edition and overflows with detailed argumentation for those wishing to dive into the philosophical deep end. Klusendorf's second edition of *The Case for Life* is one of the best single-volume books on pro-life apologetics, and it is completely accessible to someone new to the topic.

The only real connection between *Pivot* and *Contenders* is the main subject matter: abortion. *Contenders* is for those who message on bioethics (abortion, euthanasia, embryonic stem cell research, IVF, and similar topics), mainly pastors and teachers. I wrote *Pivot* for anyone who wants to save the lives of preborn children, but who may feel uncertain where their gifts, talents, and resources could best be utilized. It also serves as a resource for pastors and teachers who want a more thorough context for the problem of abortion in a post-*Roe* era where *Dobbs* sets new ground rules.

Not the Final Word

I began work on *Pivot* four years ago, though I did the bulk of the writing during the past year. Over that time, I watched the battlefield shift and change as new strategies were tried here, litigation sprang up there, and laws and constitutional amendments (both life-affirming and pro-abortion) proliferated across the political landscape.

Our opponents have not given up. They are strategic, well-funded (though recent funding restrictions have helped a bit, the ability to maintain those restrictions is in doubt), and wounded. The abortion industry has begun fighting back in ways I will expose in this book, but you can be sure they will launch other strategies and tactics. I hope that by bringing you up to speed, I may help you spot and respond to other moves by abortion advocates in every political, cultural, moral, and religious sphere where they operate.

But I want you to do more than merely respond or take a reactive approach. I hope that reading *Pivot* will spur you to adopt, adapt, or create other effective pro-life strategies. The battle over abortion is deadly serious; it's no game. Ultimately, one side or the other will win. We must develop a strategic mindset.

Although *Pivot* is not exhaustive, it is sufficient. If you've never read a comprehensive case for life, go get *Contenders* or *The Case for Life* and fill in the gaps. Then, if you and others fully implement the strategies and tactics outlined in this book, your work will go a long way toward ending the killing and creating a worldview that embraces the sanctity of human life from the cradle to the grave.

What This Book Is

Abortion divides our nation into three camps.

Some individuals in the U.S. are emotionally, politically, and financially invested in abortion. A few are spiritually devoted as well and actually *delight* in abortion. I identify and expose them in *Contenders*. There is little chance (not none, just little) of changing the minds of those who have firmly planted their flag in the abortion advocacy camp. They are committed. The only way forward is to culturally and politically defeat them.

Another section of our nation identifies themselves as committed pro-life advocates. Some of them are deeply grounded in the scientific, moral, and biblical case for life. Others feel sympathetic to protecting preborn children, even if they have not yet been taught how to defend that position. These individuals require only reinforcement.

But most Americans make up what is known as "the mushy middle." They have "leanings" and maybe even tribal loyalties, but they rarely, perhaps never, consider abortion. Instead, in blissful ignorance of the daily slaughter of more than 3,000 children, they just go about their lives. These individuals, the "persuadables," are the main target for advocacy.

Another significant group in the mushy middle is ego-involved in maintaining legal abortion because its members have participated in, or have had, abortions in their past. Nobody wants to think badly of themselves, and confronting the idea that abortion means the intentional killing of their children creates massive cognitive dissonance, which most seek to avoid. The persaudables don't care about abortion as a topic. The ego-involved don't want to think about it. To reach both the persuadable and those with an emotional connection to abortion, we need an executable plan.

"But wait!" you may object. "Haven't pro-life groups been strategizing, planning, and executing for over fifty years?" Well, yes and no. It is true that divergent groups have put programs and campaigns in motion. Most have been volunteer efforts working to dislodge a professional abortion industry that is both well-funded and in command of most of the cultural channels of national communication. Add to that the monumental legal obstacles presented by *Roe v. Wade*. That Supreme Court case not only hobbled the ability of the pro-life movement to make meaningful advances, but also muzzled many pastors, who believed that its existence made speaking about abortion a waste of precious pulpit time.

The *Dobbs* decision changed all that. Certainly, an array of pro-abortion institutions remains. But the protections on the abortion monoculture provided by *Roe* have dissolved. It's a new day. And we must prepare and take advantage of the opportunity. No one knows how long it will last, so read and act quickly.

What Lies Ahead

The first part of *Pivot* sets the stage, beginning with an overview of the impact the *Dobbs* decision had on the abortion industry. It didn't take pro-aborts by surprise; many planned ahead for a defeat they saw as inevitable. But, like the death of a beloved elderly relative, you can know it's coming and still feel rocked when it actually arrives. Predictably, pro-abortion forces lost their minds when Justice Samuel Alito's majority opinion became known. From protests to howls of derision to deranged street performances, the response looked like nothing short of a meltdown.

But only for a little while.

Pro-abortion forces, though initially staggered, retreated, then retrenched, and then came out stronger. Ultimately, the *Dobbs* decision didn't intimidate them; rather, they found ways to adapt and surge forward. Did you know that more abortions take place in the U.S. today than shortly before the overturning of *Roe*?

Part Two reveals five key pivots we need, not only to counter the advances of abortion advocates, but to take the fight for life into hostile territory. Pro-life advocates are waging a state-by-state battle for the lives of preborn children.

Pivot one lays the groundwork by showing how pro-aborts use language to shape people's understanding of abortion. It also explains how, by making a simple pivot in the way you speak, you can nullify those gains and reframe the issue.

Pivot two shows how abortion advocates use education to advance their agendas. By adopting some of the very strategies they use, you can do what they cannot: inoculate the people you teach against abortion claims. Abortion advocates can't afford to have people directly encounter a well-developed, comprehensive case for life. But pro-life advocates are unafraid. Placing the ideas promulgated by the abortion industry front and center is the first part of the strategy. Careful examination, evidenced refutation, and clear, more supportable alternatives represent the path to changes in popular attitude and action.

Pivot three explains how pro-life states haven't done enough to reinforce the life cultures of the areas they govern. A host of tactics can be employed to strengthen the knowledge and attitudes of the citizens of those states. Many of these tactics you can push to enact at the local level. If you live in a pro-life state, much of the heavy lifting is done—but it would be a mistake to rest. Enemies of life continue rattling at the gates.

And what if you live in an abortion state? Pivot four demonstrates that even though prospects for victory may seem remote, you can do a great deal. Pregnancy help centers and clinics already have established a beachhead in states hostile toward the preborn. And programs designed to move those persuadable people into supporting life-affirming legislation are being launched. So be encouraged! No matter what kind of state you live in, you have a role to fill.

Pivot five culminates in action. Throughout the book, I will reveal solutions to the problems pro-life people face in establishing protections for their preborn neighbors. In these final chapters, you will read of specific actions you can take to make some of these solutions a reality. While I have no way of knowing which roles fit which readers, be assured that there is *something* in there for *you* to do.

Expectations

I'm very glad you bought *Pivot*. If it was a gift, I hope you're glad you received it. And now, here you are—you're reading it. And though I want you to finish reading, most importantly, as with *Contenders* that preceded it, I want you to *do* it. Not everyone can do everything, but everyone can do something.

You will find a lot of "somethings" to consider as you move from chapter to chapter. It's possible to get overwhelmed and think that if you can't do it all, you may as well give up and do nothing. If such an idea should strike you, recognize it as the voice of the Enemy of your soul, whispering in your ear. Reject it.

Instead, pray, seek counsel, pick an action—maybe just a single action—that matches your gifts, skills, and/or resources. And then engage your will to do it. Now, turn the page and let's get started.

PART ONE

THE POST-*DOBBS* MELTDOWN AND MASTERPLAN

CHAPTER 1

The *Dobbs* Leak and the Doubling Down on Abortion

An angry crowd gathered outside the private home of Supreme Court Justice Brett Kavanaugh on May 2, 2022. Placards waved and bullhorns blared with the familiar call-and-response chants from abortion advocates: "No uterus, no opinion!" "My body, my choice!" and "Keep abortion safe and legal."

One of the perennial slogans required a little retrofitting. The old "Pro-life? It's a lie. You don't care if women die!" was no longer appropriate in a world where no one seems to know what a woman is. Since the protesters didn't want to be accused of erasing "trans" people, they modified the words: "Pro-life? It's a lie. You don't care if *people* die!"

The irony—that the objective of every abortion is to intentionally kill a child—was lost on the lunatics in the street.

The Supreme Court decision in *Dobbs v. Jackson Women's Health Organization* had been leaked (even today no one is sure by whom). One likely intention of the leak was to aid abortion advocates in getting out in front of the published decision, in hopes that they might be able to sway some justices and get a different outcome. But it was all for nothing. The final ruling, published less than two months later, was essentially the same as Justice Samuel Alito's leaked draft.

In a 6-3 decision, the Supreme Court overturned *Roe v. Wade*. Many pro-life advocates had so deeply desired such an outcome that they barely hoped it could happen in their lifetime. And suddenly, it became reality. The clock reset to 1973 and individual states could once again craft their own abortion legislation without interference from the federal government. In some states, trigger laws protecting preborn children immediately went into effect. While the ruling wounded abortion rights advocates, it hardly defeated them. Like a predator whose territory has been violated, the abortion industry immediately lashed out.

In this chapter, I'll begin by revealing some of the targeted messaging pro-aborts unleashed after the *Dobbs* decision dropped, including direct and indirect attacks on pregnancy help centers and clinics. Then I'll expose the truly unhinged behavior that can be expected of those who believe it is their right to intentionally kill children in the womb, and the disappointing response of many churches. Finally, you'll see how the abortion industry pivoted, including their strategy to flip pro-life states.

Abortion Advocates Respond to Dobbs

In addition to mobs screaming outside of Supreme Court justices' homes following the *Dobbs* decision leak, protests immediately erupted across the country. No longer did abortion advocates hide behind verbiage such as "pro-choice" or the idea that "abortion should be safe, legal, and rare." Instead, banners featured aggressive slogans such as "Abortion on Demand Without Apology," "Rise Up 4 Abortion Rights" and "Defend Abortion Rights by Any Means Necessary." Crowds chanting "Abortion Rights are Human Rights" and "Keep your rosaries off my ovaries" filled the streets of major American cities.[2]

Memes erupted on social media, fueling fears that overturning *Roe* would lead to dire consequences. Posts warned that the *Dobbs* decision would lead to women dying from ectopic pregnancies and "septic uterus."

Physicians would refuse to deliver stillborn children, leading inevitably to a massive rise in maternal deaths. Women *must* have abortion, citizens were told, because pregnancy is unacceptably dangerous. Without *Roe*, the apocalypse was upon us.

In states banning abortion post-*Dobbs*, Americans heard that women would die. Maternal mortality rates would skyrocket. Indeed, some studies reported that states with more restrictions on abortion had a higher rate of adverse outcomes not only for women, but for babies, because of a higher perinatal death rate (this includes children who die within four weeks of birth) in restrictive states.[3]

The pattern in James 1:14-16 is clear: lust leads to sin, and sin ends in death. That pattern is borne out in abortion, but also in the reaction of committed abortion activists to any attempt to protect preborn children.

Abortion supporters denigrated pro-life advocates, not as pro-life, but as pro-"forced birth." Who would oppose abortion, they wondered? Only misogynistic controllers of women's bodies, they answered. Some called pro-life advocates hypocritical because they did not support gun control legislation.[4] By linking the term "forced"—a "devil term" if ever there was one in the freedom-loving U.S.—with the word "birth," the user connected something repulsive (who likes being forced?) with a word generally considered positive. The goal? To make readers reject "pro-life" people and politicians as purveyors of unwanted, unsafe forced births.

Beyond creating fear of maternal deaths and raising the specter of an impending real-life *Handmaid's Tale*, abortion advocates wanted to generate sympathy and pity for a "need" for late-term abortion. Without legal abortion, they cried, women would be forced (there's that word again) to give birth to children with severe or fatal fetal deformities. In some states, life protection laws did not include exceptions for rape and incest; and pro-aborts asserted that only a moral monster would require a victim of sexual assault to give birth to the perpetrator's baby.

No Competing Narratives Allowed

The media gives wide coverage to the views of abortion advocates, often joined by the public education system. Nearly every national-level policy-maker in the Democratic Party lauds such views, the American College of Obstetricians and Gynecologists endorses them, and even the pulpits of some churches proclaim them. But despite the cultural near-monopoly of their message, abortion proponents remain unsatisfied. A major source of their discontent is the continued existence of what they repeatedly call "crisis pregnancy centers."

It didn't take the *Dobbs* decision to cause state agencies to vilify Pregnancy Help Centers and Clinics (PHCs). The mere existence of these "abortion alternative" organizations posed an existential threat. If abortion really is a woman's right and a key aspect of fundamental health care, then any individual or organization that claimed abortion was wrong for women and children should be stripped of its voice. Abortion advocacy states and organizations would much prefer that PHCs not exist at all. Abortion states thus did what they could to push PHCs to the margins.

California

The State of California hosts an official website directing pregnant women to abortion facilities. On the page "California Abortion Access," the state informs pregnant women (or men who want to direct their pregnant "partner") that "Abortion remains safe, legal, and accessible in California, whether or not you live in the state."[5] It then details "abortion steps," "types of abortion," and "how to pay."[6]

None of the entries describing abortion types reference in any way the presence of the child in the womb. The explanation of a "medication abortion" (using the abortion pill) never identifies exactly *what* (actually *who*) is being eliminated. In the section on "In-clinic procedures," the closest the state comes to telling the reader about the *target* of the removal "procedure" describes the child as "pregnancy tissue."[7]

Unsure about where to find an abortionist? The State of California is happy to help. By partnering with Abortion Finder, anyone can locate the nearest abortion facility. It's important to the state that the reader finds only *abortion* facilities, so it includes a section called "Fake Abortion Information," where it identifies "crisis pregnancy centers" as villains. It also supplies a direct link to Planned Parenthood's alarming article, "Crisis Pregnancy Centers: What to Know and How to Spot Them."[8]

Why are pregnancy help centers and clinics identified as the nemesis of Planned Parenthood? It's because PHCs reveal what Planned Parenthood, and other abortion industry allies, would like to hide: that abortion intentionally kills innocent children in the womb. In order to divert pregnant women away from PHCs, Planned Parenthood offers the following as a description:

> Crisis pregnancy centers (also called CPCs or "fake clinics") are clinics or mobile vans that look like real health centers, but they're run by anti-abortion activists who have a shady, harmful agenda: to scare, shame, or pressure you out of getting an abortion, and to tell lies about abortion, birth control, and sexual health... Crisis pregnancy centers don't provide abortion or offer a full range of health care, and they won't give you honest facts about sexual health and your pregnancy options—their goal is to spread misinformation and propaganda.[9]

The State of California also links to a state Justice Department PDF that it claims will show readers "how to spot fake clinics."[10] In the eyes of

California, the only legitimate "reproductive health clinics" are those that not only discourage reproduction but that also advocate for, and engage in, the intentional killing of children, the results of reproduction. And if you can't afford your elective abortion, the site is happy to direct you to organizations that will help pay to end your child's life.

Sadly, California is hardly alone in using official web pages to promote abortion. The following are a few additional examples.

Oregon

The Oregon Health Authority page opens with an attempt to "normalize" abortion, telling readers that "about one in four people in the US who can become pregnant will have an abortion by age 45."[11] Oregon also partners with Abortion Finder, the National Abortion Federation, and with Reproductive Health Access (which provides Oregon's "Where to Get an Abortion" page[12] with a link to its own "How to Spot and Avoid Fake Abortion Clinics"[13]).

Washington State

Not to be outdone, the Washington State Department of Health page comes complete with an exit button, just in case someone sees you looking at a state-sponsored web page about abortion.[14] It makes it clear that abortion is available to all, regardless of residency. One web page offers a step-by-step guide to Plan for Your Abortion.[15]

The last thing Washington State wants anyone to do is to interact with PHCs, so it has a big, clickable button to take visitors to the "Avoid Anti-Abortion Facilities" page.[16] There viewers will encounter a bulleted list of allegations designed to alarm the reader. The claims are just vague enough to shield the state from civil suits, using words such as "most," "usually," "sometimes," and "may." The page makes it clear that, according to Washington State, the only legitimate health care facilities are those that either perform or refer for abortions. No other narratives are allowed.

Additional States

Other states with dedicated pro-abortion sites include New York, Minnesota, New Jersey, Maine, and New Mexico.[17] The desire to eradicate any narrative but their own, however, is not limited to pro-abortion state governments. Private citizens, sometimes acting alone and at other times collectively, and emboldened by the rhetoric of national organizations and inflamed by the idea that their cherished "abortion rights" were under siege, also have acted out.

Arson, Vandalism, and Assault

Once the official educational and state mouthpieces declared the "dangers" posed by PHCs, it didn't take long for some individuals to conclude that such "fake clinics" must be silenced and destroyed. Following the *Dobbs* decision, PHCs were firebombed, covered with graffiti, and their employees threatened and harassed.

The Family Research Council published a PDF containing links to nearly forty attacks on churches, sixty-seven attacks on pregnancy centers and pro-life organizations, and twenty-four other examples of assault, vandalism, graffiti and more—all occurring within a year of the May 2, 2022 leak of the *Dobbs* decision.[18] St. Joseph's Church in Michigan was defaced with a spray-painted pentagram, the number 666, vulgarities and death threats. The doors of Sacred Heart of Mary, a Catholic church in Boulder, Colorado, were painted with abortion slogans: "My body, my choice" and "Bans off our bodies."

An arson fire engulfed a pregnancy resource center in Gresham, Oregon, when perpetrators threw Molotov cocktails through the window.[19] CompassCare Pregnancy Services in Amherst, New York, had to hire a private investigator and file FACE Act charges when the FBI failed to investigate an arson attack that significantly damaged the center in June 2022. Five other centers were victims of arson; all their cases remain unsolved.[20] Centers faced intimidation, some spray-painteddirectly on the walls of their buildings, often including variants of the threat "If abortion isn't safe, neither are you," sometimes accompanied by "Jane's Revenge."[21] Many centers had to deal with broken windows, increased security costs, and disruption to their ministry to women seeking life-affirming alternatives to abortion.

College and university campuses, once bastions of free speech, have become sites of violent intolerance toward any student or group voicing pro-life messages. At Kent State University in 2024, a display of crosses, representing the number of children whose lives were lost to abortion in Ohio, proved too much for abortion advocates. They ripped up the crosses and tore down pro-life signage.[22] Pro-life displays on campuses, designed to be a point of engagement with students, are routinely spray-painted, vandalized, or destroyed.

Despite the attacks, PHCs and advocacy groups continue their work unabated. Heather Vasquez, executive director of Next Step Pregnancy Services in Washington (a center that had windows broken and was spray painted) provided photos of the damage for me, accompanied by this response:

> We stayed open that day and every day since then. As you can see, one of our folks worked on the door and our supporters helped repair windows. We kept the spray on the back wall. And I kept the rock that flew through my window as a reminder. We stayed open. We were not deterred. Clients came anyway. Most were shocked and saddened and above all confused as to why we were targeted.
>
> I remember feeling determined. Angry. Resolute. And proud. Proud to be chosen by God for this battle in this place at this time. Still do.[23]

Every center director I spoke with after the attacks felt the same way. They remained uniformly unbowed, unbroken, and humbled to be a part of such a significant work.

Abortion Advocates Unhinged

Think for a moment about the natural effect that decades of legalized abortion must have on any nation that practices it. The very idea that loud, proud advocates of intentionally killing children in the womb could feel free to parade their view in public in a civilized nation boggles the mind. But exist they do, examples of what the Apostle Paul describes in the first chapter of Romans: those who do not "see fit to acknowledge God any longer, [so] God gave them over to a depraved mind."[24]

Ayman Mohyeldin led a discussion, following the *Dobbs* leak, on his MSNBC News show. One of the panelists, comedian Laurie Kilmartin, commented:

> Here's my feeling about the leaker. I would like to find out who the leaker is, so I could make sweet love to that person, because that person is a hero to me. Okay? And if the leaker—a lot of people are saying it could be a conservative—if the leaker is a Republican, and if I get pregnant during our lovemaking, I will joyfully abort our fetus, and let them know.[25]

Instead of being horrified, Mohyeldin and fellow panelists, Joan Walsh and Maria Teresa Kumar, simply laughed.

Laughter in response to discussions about the intentional killing of children in the womb is not limited to television personalities who enjoy the protection of a supportive network. Unfortunately, it's nothing new. At a meeting of abortion practitioners held in San Francisco in 2014, an undercover operative for The Center for Medical Progress recorded Uta

Landy, founder of Consortium of Abortion Providers (CAPS) and the first executive director of the National Abortion Federation, reciting comments that she had received from abortionists: "...and another, 'An eyeball just fell into my lap, and it was gross!' (prolonged laughter from the audience of abortion providers). 'But I say to myself, this abortion is going well, and is going safely, so I am fine.' (more laughter).[26]

Days after the *Dobbs* leak, in New York City, a female performance "artist" going by the name Crackhead Barney led a pro-abortion protest to the steps of the Basilica of St. Patrick's Old Cathedral. Wearing a threadbare one-piece swimsuit, she simulated giving birth by pulling out multiple baby dolls, which had been stuffed into her suit, out of the leg opening. The dolls were connected by a pink cloth representing the umbilical cord. She then slammed the dolls' heads on the concrete while screaming, "I'm killing the babies! I'm killing the babies!"

A couple of years later, a street interviewer asked "Crackhead Barney" what "she wants people to feel when they watch her videos." She replied: "I want people to vomit...I want people to be disgusted by me. That's really the main point."[27]

Mission accomplished.

Something else, however, should disturb those who still have a clear moral compass. Why would anyone choose to be "entertained" by someone gleefully engaging in imitation infanticide on a public street? To their credit, a group of Catholic men stood vigil outside the basilica, not engaging the protestors directly, but instead praying.

Church Reactions

Despite the hysterical rhetoric on social media, the response of pro-abortion states and the abortion industry, the vandalism and violence, and the unhinged voices in the news and on the streets, one might hope that at least the Church—the one cultural voice purportedly dedicated to God's

Word, proclaiming truth, and rejoicing in justice—would celebrate a rare, unified moment of cultural victory.

Dobbs provided a path forward for Christian voices to succeed at saving the lives of preborn children, created in the image of God, from the threat of abortion. And now not only through PHCs, but in the law. However, just as the church was divided on abortion during the *Roe* era, so that division continues today.

For one side, the *Dobbs* decision did not provide the outright victory desired. Abortion states were still free to operate abortion facilities and kill preborn children. Federal protection for children in the womb did not exist. Under *Roe*, states wanting to protect preborn children were shackled by the Supreme Court decision. But now, under *Dobbs*, those same states are free to enact safeguards. It's not the total victory pro-life advocates wanted, but it is still a significant advance.

Children remain at risk from abortion today only because the citizens of some states want it. At the same time, these same citizens are free at any time to protect those children. Persuasion can lead to effective life-saving campaigns. While *Dobbs* was a titanic step forward in the fight for life, you'd be hard-pressed to notice it in some churches.

Some pastors cautioned their parishioners not to openly celebrate the greatest opportunity to stand in the gap for preborn lives that most of them had ever experienced. Phil Metzger, pastor of Calvary San Diego, said:

> There's a whole group of people that don't see today as a victory, they see it as a huge loss, and I don't have to kind of rub that in on anybody like, "Oh yay for this," because I don't want to demonize people that have had to make the hard choice of having an abortion... It's a reality that when one domino falls we go how many other dominoes are about to fall. So I get the fear that certain communities in our state and country feel.[28]

It's not hard to find examples of similar sentiments. [29]

What should have been a nationwide celebration to rival the Emancipation Proclamation or one of the major victories of WWII, instead in some churches became a cautious, muted response to "keep it down." After the Emancipation Proclamation and at the end of the Civil War, you could almost hear such pastors saying, "Be gracious, everyone. A lot of people lost their property today." The lack of scientific, moral, and biblical insight and standards in such churches astonishes me.

Unbeaten

Following the leak of *Dobbs*, and especially after publication of the final ruling, the abortion industry went into full meltdown mode. Protests, narrative lockdowns, physical violence, and all manner of grotesque acting out – abortion advocates were experiencing an existential crisis – but only for a moment. Even some churches couldn't celebrate, and their overcautiousness dampened what should have been battle cry. For the first time in five decades, the way had been cleared of the impediment of *Roe*. States could finally protect preborn children from those who would intentionally kill them. But the opponents of life weren't beaten; they barely took a pause.

The Abortion Industry Pivots, Too

All the breathless claims of concern by abortion advocates, the abortion industry, and their shock troops and media mouthpieces ignored the fact that in a post-*Roe* America, abortion continued unabated in most states. Prior to the *Dobbs* decision, some states already had constitutional barriers in place guaranteeing a right to elective abortion just in case *Roe* was overturned.

In Kansas, for example, a State Supreme Court case in 2019 ruled that the state constitution protected abortion to the degree that any moves to limit some kinds of abortion, or to eliminate or restrain abortion coordinated through the internet, are legally enjoined.[30] After *Dobbs*, other states passed constitutional amendments to guarantee abortion rights. Some, such as Colorado, allowed for abortion throughout pregnancy, while others, such as Arizona, appeared to leave some meager viability restrictions in place while including broad exceptions for physical and mental health that, practically speaking, eliminate any meaningful restrictions.

Other states without constitutional protection continued their abortion business under statute law. North Carolina, for example, had some pro-life protections in place; but provisions such as a twelve-week ban don't do much to stop the killing of preborn children, as approximately 90 percent of elective abortions take place before the restriction kicks in.

Abortion Expansion in Process

Most of the pearl-clutching rhetoric came from pro-abortion organizations, politicians, and advocates, many of whom live and work in states where abortion is currently legal and protected. But abortion-industry workers and apologists are not satisfied to merely live in abortion states. They want to destroy any group or organization inside their state that would dare to offer a competing narrative.

With the zeal of immoral evangelists, they cannot rest until every state in the union has abortion on demand, for any reason whatsoever, at taxpayer expense—and if the mother is a minor, without parental knowledge or consent. If they can't get taxpayers to foot the bill, plenty of others remain so committed that they willingly donate their own hard-earned cash and services to make it possible to abort more children.

Abortion Funds

Since air travel has become increasingly burdensome, I prefer to drive whenever I can. Not only can I stop whenever I want, but I can get a steak for dinner at a Texas Roadhouse just off the interstate, instead of getting pelted with pretzels from a well-meaning flight attendant. Driving also educates me in local political battles represented by roadside billboards.

Cruising through Wyoming on my way to speak, I came upon a sign for Chelsea's Fund. I'm used to seeing funds for lots of things. My parents used to donate to the Christian Children's Fund. When you want to give online to someone in need, there is GoFundMe. These funds are designed to help people in need. But Chelsea's Fund collects money to facilitate the intentional killing of children in the womb by providing for travel expenses, lodging, or even paying for the recipient's abortion.[31] I'd never seen such a thing before.

Chelsea's Fund is no outlier. These "charities" are so numerous they have their own clearinghouse, The National Network of Abortion Funds.[32] They represent nearly 100 separate groups dedicated to giving money to moms who want to end their children's lives. One of their recent press releases championed their desire to help minors exercise their "bodily autonomy."[33]

As chapters three and four explain, chemical abortions can reach anywhere in the U.S. Only if the child in the womb reaches a certain gestational age is the abortion pill not advised (and, as you will discover, that gestational age limit continues to expand). So then, what happens if that mother lives in a state with a Human Life Protection Act, and the age of her developing child means that only a surgical abortion is indicated? What if she can't afford transportation costs, or car travel would be too troublesome? Abortion advocates have her covered. Elevated Access will help fly her to her abortion destination.

'Abortion Air'

Elevated Access has more than 700 pilots available to whisk people from pro-life states to abortion states. They also transport teenagers to states where they can access transgender hormone services. The founder, who just goes by "Mike," says he knows that many major corporations provide abortion travel to their employees living in states with life-affirming laws.

Flying, a website dedicated to aviation enthusiasts, explains how Elevated Access found its niche: "According to Mike, however, employees of large companies aren't the demographic most affected by the recent ruling nor are they the neediest."[34] And so there now exists an "Abortion Air" service, explicitly identified as a response to *Dobbs*, that *Flying* compares to aviation support for "medical care" or "animal rescue." *Rolling Stone* breathlessly referred to Elevated Access as an "airlift."

Odd that these publications would compare Elevated Access to medical care, animal rescue, or an "airlift," a word often associated with getting people out of a war zone, rather than taking people to a place where they can intentionally kill another human being.[35]

The abortion industry is willing to do whatever it takes to keep performing abortions, and not just where they legally can, but everywhere. Workarounds don't satisfy abortion advocates. The very existence of pregnancy centers and life protection laws acts as a living indictment of their worldview, so they work hard to flip pro-life states so that legal abortion will, once again, be the law of the land.

The Handbook for Overturning Pro-Life Protections

Robin Marty wrote one of the most popular instruction manuals outlining the plans of abortion advocates, titled *Handbook for a Post-Roe America*. Originally written in 2019 and updated two years later, Marty was gearing up for an increase in laws protecting the lives of preborn children even before the *Dobbs* decision. Imagining an America without legal abortion, Marty revised her book to respond to the "ways advocates [of abortion] and pregnant people will be forced to adapt if abortion is made partially or completely illegal in the United States" and "what would be needed if legal abortion clinics truly ceased to exist..."[36]

Violate the Law

The updates included strategies such as engaging in civil disobedience, transporting women and minors from pro-life states to abortion states, vetting doctors to see who would be willing to violate any restrictions or bans on abortion, and instructions on how women can perform abortions on themselves at home. Not long ago, one of the rallying images used by abortion advocates was a coat hanger, designed to evoke the picture of an ugly crone in an attic somewhere wielding a rusty wire as an abortion tool on unsuspecting, desperate women. Worse yet, the distraught woman might use the coat hanger on herself. Legal abortion was necessary, the idea went, to keep women from engaging unqualified people to perform an abortion or to keep pregnant women from DIY abortions.

Not only was the use of such imagery insulting to women, it wasn't remotely accurate. Back when abortion was illegal, abortions may have been performed in "the back alley," but it was the alley that led to a doctor's office, the site of many illegal abortions. Even prior to *Roe*, abortion advocates admitted that even illegal abortions were safe for women.[37] But in her book, Marty offers instruction on self-induced aspiration abortions as well as an herbal guide. Abortion advocacy, it appears, has abandoned the need for doctors. It now encourages pregnant women to perform abortion on themselves, or women without medical training to perform them on each other.

Leverage Selective Pity to Change the Law

Marty recommends an appeal to selective pity to undermine and overturn every single life protection law in all pro-life states. She writes:

> Pressuring your legislators to ensure that at a minimum victims of sexual assault still have access to abortion care—and aren't forced to carry to term just because of the state they live in—is not just a reasonable action that reflects the majority's belief on abortion. It also offers a clear incremental step toward repealing abortion bans as a whole down the road, and it exposes just how radical the Right's position has become.[38]

Marty suggests that abortion advocates use circumstances such as rape and incest as a strategy to overturn any type of life-affirming legislation. Notice how she characterizes a woman's pregnancy: "forced to carry to term" instead of recognizing that her body is performing a natural and good function: protecting and nurturing her child. Her book demonstrates that she would not be satisfied with rape and incest exceptions embedded in otherwise pro-life legislation. She would reject such legislation for the same reason that pro-life legislators should not include them.

Abortion advocates implicitly understand that any exception to full abortion on demand means there are at least some circumstances under which abortion should not be allowed. They only argue for rape and incest exceptions as stepping stones. Their reasoning being: if it is morally permissible to kill children because of the circumstances of their conception, then preborn children aren't really sacrosanct, and there may be a host of other circumstances that would also justify putting them to death. When pro-life legislators include rape and incest exceptions, they provide tacit approval for this line of thinking. The only excuse for using any kinds of exceptions is because it may not be politically tenable, at present, to push for other protections without them. But the goal must always be to use the newly-captured ground as a platform from which to press on for Human Life Protection Acts which ban abortion, without exceptions.

Push Back

What do you do when your opponents are committed? Abortion advocates are willing to give of their time, their talents, and their financial resources to intentionally end the lives of preborn children. They support, think, and strategize about abortion. To them, abortion isn't just a passing political issue that requires attention every two to four years, it is an existential part of their lives.

The internet, airwaves, and lecture halls of America are awash with pro-abortion rhetoric. Your voice, and the voices of many others, are needed to push back, building protective walls to safeguard your preborn neighbors. In the next chapter, I'll analyze and provide responses to a few of these arguments that gained more traction in the wake of *Dobbs*.

CHAPTER 2

Cruel and Fatal Accusations

How should pro-life advocates respond to recent advances made by the abortion industry? What can opponents of intentional child-killing say to counter the rape and incest arguments of pro-aborts? And what should we make of "forced birth" claims as reasons for killing children in the womb?

In this chapter I'll reveal and analyze the rape and incest exception arguments, then do the same with the lies spread by popular social media memes after *Dobbs*. Finally, I'll unpack the pro-abortion idea that if their arguments are rejected, the only remaining position for pro-life advocates is "forced birth."

Rape and Incest Exceptions

Robin Marty, the author of *Handbook for a Post-Roe America*, knows that rape and incest exceptions undermine the philosophical basis for rejecting abortion as a whole. Exception arguments move the focus of legislation away from who is being protected (children in the womb) and toward the circumstances of conception.

Exception arguments aren't the last step in legislation offered by abortion advocates, but merely the first. If abortion advocates can get voters to believe that it is morally permissible to intentionally kill children if they were conceived through a criminal act, then they have at least one circumstance in which it is morally permissible to kill children. And if one exception is permitted, why not others?

Exceptions Multiply

If a child can be intentionally killed in the womb because she was conceived through rape, then why can't a child be killed because the mother lost her job or her partner?[39] There is no bright-line distinction during pregnancy, in Marty's analysis, that says people can intentionally kill their children for some reasons, but not others. Instead, she invites voters to consider one reason why it would be okay, and then she would extend that single exception to additional life events. Once legislative focus shifts from the target of abortion—the preborn child—to the life circumstances of the mother, *any* reason for abortion becomes acceptable.

Selective Pity

Exception arguments are the strategy, but the tactic employed to achieve the goal is selective pity. Marty knows that people rightfully view rape as a horrific crime, a sexual violation of a woman's body. The rapist is a criminal. The female target is a victim. The criminal should be punished and the victim deserves pity.

But according to Marty's assessment, the *only* victim in view is the woman. Not a single thought is offered for the innocent child growing in the mother's womb. Doesn't that child—also a victim, also a casualty of circumstance—also deserve pity?

How can Christians navigate these arguments? We can do so by distinguishing between the action of pity and the passion of pity, best explained by C.S. Lewis in *The Great Divorce*. Lewis describes a bus ride from hell's suburbs to the outskirts of heaven, where sinners are offered a final chance to turn from their sins. Almost all the passengers refuse to repent, preferring to return to "the Grey Town" rather than embrace the offer and enter the heavenly realm.

In one passage, the protagonist, who has come up from the Grey Town, meets with Lewis' real-life hero and mentor, George MacDonald. Together, they witness a citizen of heaven meet her former husband who has arrived on the bus. He has always used appeals to his wretchedness and misery to compel the woman to do his ungodly will, but that strategy doesn't work in heaven.

MacDonald explains to the protagonist that appeals to pity, once analyzed, often amount to nothing more than some individuals pressuring others into agreeing with what is evil so they can avoid causing the "offended" person discomfort. It can be used as a weapon to gain concessions from good people. An extreme example would be the man who kills his own parents and then throws himself on the mercy of the court because he is, after all, a pitiful orphan. MacDonald argues that in heaven, pity must die. The man replies:

> "But dare one say—it is horrible to say—that Pity must die?"
>
> "Ye must distinguish. The action of Pity will live forever, but the passion of Pity will not. The Passion of pity, the pity we merely suffer, the ache that draws men to concede what should not be conceded and to flatter when they should speak truth, the pity that has cheated many a woman out of her virginity and many a statesman out of his honesty—that will die. It was used as a weapon by bad men against good ones: their weapon will be broken."
>
> "And what is the other kind—the action?"
>
> "It is a weapon on the other side [the side of good]. It leaps quicker than light from the highest place to the lowest to bring healing and

> joy, whatever the cost to itself. It changes darkness into light and evil into good. But it will not, at the cunning tears of Hell, impose on good the tyranny of evil. Every disease that submits to a cure shall be cured: but we will not call blue yellow to please those who insist on still having jaundice nor make a midden [a dung heap] of the world's garden for the sake of some who cannot abide the smell of roses."[40]

In the abortion debate, many arguments that appeal to circumstances, such as conditions of conception (rape or incest), economic or relational issues, and others, are appeals to the passion of pity. Those making such claims want you to forget that the act of abortion kills an innocent preborn human being. They want you to focus, instead, on the distress or discomfort of the woman experiencing an untimely pregnancy.

In other cases, the object of misplaced pity is a man who perceives he will be negatively impacted by the birth of his own child. Pete Buttigieg, after losing the Democratic Party nomination for president, expressed just that sentiment during a fundraising event for White Dudes for Kamala:

> I'm so glad she has made freedom the theme of her campaign, and I think in so many ways that's what's at stake. And, yes, women's freedom is Exhibit A after Donald Trump demolished the right to choose. But, of course, men are also more free in a country where we have a president who stands up for things like access to abortion care.[41]

Passion of Pity Dangers

Rape and incest are horrific crimes and those perpetrating them, if convicted, should be punished to the full extent of the law. The victim of such a crime, however, is entirely innocent and is worthy of all the aid and support she requires. She *should* receive the action of pity. Similarly, because the preborn child is likewise innocent, she should not be cruelly put to death. She should not be given over to an abortionist who will violate her bodily integrity even more violently than the rapist did her mother. The child should, like the mother, receive the action of pity.

Other arguments that presume the preborn children aren't human beings, or simply dismiss their existence altogether, want the listener to feel the passion of pity *only* for the woman who finds herself in difficult circumstances.

But the circumstances of the woman can change. What she values can change. Her desires and dreams can change. Caring people can rally around her and help her to find the physical, emotional, and spiritual help she needs. But *no one* should use the passion of pity to convince her that because she was violated, she should now conspire to kill her preborn child. Neither should she use that passion to convince herself that she'd be morally justified to snuff out the life of her son or daughter living in her womb.

Instead, the action of pity should move us all to protect the life of the child endangered by those who would deny or dismiss her so they might kill her. What people in distress need is not the *passion* of pity, but the *action* of pity, coupled with the grace to endure.

Responding to Emboldened Pro-Abortion Advocates

Part Two of this book will deal with strategies and tactics designed to defeat the abortion industry, but right now I want to respond to the "arguments" (such as they are) that arose during the period just before and after *Dobbs*.

The Memes

Immediately following the *Dobbs* decision, my social media feed overflowed with memes describing in apocalyptic terms what American women could now expect. The fear appeals, both abundant and horrifying, came pouring in:

- Women *en masse* would die from ectopic pregnancy
- Women would die from miscarriages leading to "septic uterus" (not the correct term, but they meant that life-threatening sepsis would afflict women who miscarried and doctors would refuse to deliver the dead child, for fear of prosecution)
- Abortion on demand must be enshrined in the law

All of this was a lie, based on a lack of information guided by a devious rhetorical strategy.

Lying About Ectopic Pregnancies

Not a single state in the U.S. would prohibit a doctor from treating a woman carrying an ectopic pregnancy. In vanishingly rare cases, children who develop outside of the womb do manage to come to term, be delivered, and live.

Suze Lopez, a California nurse, unknowingly carried her child, who was growing in her abdomen but was obscured by a twenty-two-pound ovarian cyst.[42] Dr. John Ozimek, the medical director of Labor and Delivery at the Cedars-Sinai hospital where the child was delivered, estimated that the odds of such successful development and birth are less "than one in a million."[43]

A full ninety-nine percent of ectopic pregnancies occur inside one of the mother's fallopian tubes. It is not possible, at this stage of our medical technology, to transplant the embryonic child from the fallopian tube to the uterus. The longer the child develops there, the greater the chance that the fallopian tube will rupture, leading to death for the child and life-threatening complications for the mother. The child cannot gestate successfully there and will, under all circumstances, die. Therefore, the doctor will either inject methotrexate to stop cell division in the embryonic child, surgically remove the embryo, or remove the fallopian tube containing the child. The goal of the treatment is to save the life of the mother, knowing that nothing can be done to preserve the life of her child.

Dobbs opponents implied that restrictions on abortion would mean that treatment for ectopic pregnancy would be outlawed because it would be considered an abortion. But the definition of "elective abortion" is the *intentional* killing of a preborn child, and treating ectopic pregnancies does not fit that definition. In every instance of treatment for ectopic pregnancy, the death of the preborn child certainly is *foreseen* but not *intended*. The child will die if the mother is treated or not. But the death of the child is not the *purpose* of the treatment.

Misinformed About Miscarriage Management

The second fear appeal claims that women experiencing miscarriage could not get abortions designed to save their lives. The most famous case cited is that of Texas resident Amanda Zurawski, whose heart-wrenching testimony at a congressional hearing in 2023 became the rationale for abortion advocates to overturn life protection laws.[44] Zurawski was eighteen weeks pregnant when her water broke. Testimony shows that physicians, thought to be intimidated by Texas' prohibition on abortion when a heartbeat can be detected, waited until the child was dead before removing her, leading to sepsis in the mother, a life-threatening condition.

What happened to Zurawski was unbelievably tragic. No one should have to suffer as she did. But the answer to Zurawski's predicament is not to reinstate abortion on demand. Dr. Ingrid Skop, board-certified OB/GYN, testifying in the same hearing, explained the standard of care Zurawski's doctors should have followed:

> Amanda, I want to say that I'm so sorry at your loss of Willow, and I'm so sorry that your doctors misunderstood Texas law. I reviewed Texas law, of course, because I practice there and I want to understand, as well as all of the other laws in the states. Every single law allows an exclusion for a doctor to use their reasonable medical judgment to determine when to intervene in a medical emergency, which is usually defined as a threat to the life of the mother

> or permanent irreversible damage to an organ or an organ system. None of the states have the terminology that the threat must be immediate...The American College of Obstetrics and Gynecology in regards to the horrible situation that Amanda found herself in—pre-viable premature rupture of membranes where the water bag breaks, but labor does not ensue and the baby is a long way from being able to live outside of the mother. The American College acknowledges that the risk of infection is high, which can become sepsis, which can threaten the mother's life. The likelihood that the baby can make it to an age in which it can live is very low, and they tell us, and obstetricians do follow ACOG's recommendations for the standard of care. They tell us at the time of diagnosis that we should offer immediate termination of pregnancy, which they define as induction, or dilation and evacuation abortion, or expectant management. So, in a woman who is not currently infected and sick, I have had patients who have wanted to stay pregnant in hopes that they could get the baby to a gestational age where it could live, but it has always been the standard of care and continues to be the standard of care to offer delivery at that time. Most of my patients have opted for induction rather than D&E because they wanted to have a baby to mourn, but either one could have been offered and should have been offered to Amanda.[45]

Then, Dr. Skop explained why these doctors failed Ms. Zurawski:

> I think that what's going on on the ground in Texas, and I will agree with Dr. Verma and Ms. Zurawski, there is confusion. Normally, doctors, of course, are not legally trained and normally they depend on advice from their professional societies to help them understand new laws. What has been noticeably absent in Texas is any statement from the Texas Medical Association, any statement from the Texas Board of Medicine, Board of Pharmacy, Board of Nursing,

> Hospital Association, so all of these organizations, you can figure out why they might be silent. Make your own conclusions, but they have been silent.[46]

What can prevent the kind of harrowing medical emergency that Amanda Zurawski experienced? It's not abortion on demand. It is education. Specifically, doctors must be reminded by their legal teams and professional associations what the law in fact allows. Physicians should never fear prosecution for engaging in life-saving treatment. Mandated, continuing education for medical professionals, and the legal teams that advise them, would solve this problem.

The 'Forced Birth' Accusation

"You're not pro-life, you're just forced birth!" This charge against pro-life advocates has been around for many years, but social media feeds exploded with the accusation following *Dobbs*. An *ad hominem* attack—against pro-life advocates as persons—it frames the issue this way: "You don't care about women or their lives; you are interested only in compelling a woman, against her will, to carry an undesired pregnancy to term and to give birth to a child she doesn't even want." The unstated conclusion is that only patriarchal misogynists compelled to control women's bodies would do such a thing.

Another example of this kind of argument goes like this: "If your pro-life commitment doesn't extend to a wide array of other favored policy issues, then you can't authentically claim to be pro-life." In this rhetorical world, to be "authentically" pro-life would require you to be in favor of gun control, free school lunches, free housing, all clean water and air initiatives (no matter how intrusive), free contraception, etc. A bit later you'll read about a Planned Parenthood representative who argued in Senate testimony that opposing abortion itself is "anti-life."

Rational Responses

Here's the standard (and rational) pro-life response: Who gets to define what constitutes pro-life? If you did all of the things that people making the forced birth claim wanted you to do, would they then join you in eradicating the intentional killing of children in the womb? What effect would engaging in every endeavor have on the main issue? How does lack of support for a federal housing program make intentionally killing children in the womb morally permissible? I might add that many organizations already specialize in all of the other desired policy ideas (and they go after them with a singular focus), so why is it unacceptable for one organization to exist which concentrates solely on strategies to stop the killing?

> The easiest way to lose a debate is to allow your opponent to define terms. When people accept language about children in the womb that causes them to think of blobs, tumors, or parasites, the battle is lost.

Andrew Harris, a communication professor at Cedarville University, suggested a better approach. In conversation (I was teaching a pro-life public speaking class at Cedarville as the *Dobbs* decision was handed down) he explained that, in fact, it's abortion advocates who actually favor "forced birth." Follow the reasoning here.

How do you define "birth"? Birth occurs when something that is on the inside develops and transitions to the outside. If you are talking about the birth of an idea, for example, you imagine someone who's thought through a process or imagined the development of a product, and then worked to see that vision through until it becomes a tangible reality. Regarding childbirth, a child develops in the womb of his or her mother and then, when the time is right, the child transitions from inside the womb to join the rest of the world outside.

All pregnancies end in one of three ways: through natural miscarriage or stillbirth; through intentional, elective abortion; or through live birth. In two instances, no force is applied. In a miscarriage or stillbirth, the child dies of natural causes. No external force ends the life of that child. In live birth, the child completes his or her developmental stages in the womb and then is delivered into the mother's waiting arms. (Even in a Caesarean birth, an opening is created for the child to emerge. Most people wouldn't call that being "forced.")

Only during an elective abortion are lethal drugs ingested to intentionally cut off life-sustaining nutrition and hydration from the child. A second drug is then administered to force the uterus to contract, prematurely expelling the child. Alternatively, surgical instruments are forcibly inserted into the womb (the cervix has to be artificially, forcefully dilated, because in its natural state during a healthy pregnancy it closes tightly in order to protect the developing child). Finally, the child is violently dismembered and pulled from the uterus in pieces. In these cases, the child is forcibly "birthed" through a brutal act designed to unnaturally remove the child's body from the womb to the outside world, where it will be disposed of as medical waste.

The pregnant woman is carrying a child. The child's natural location is inside the mother's uterus. No one is "compelling her" to be pregnant; she naturally is pregnant. There is nothing immoral about a law preventing people from intentionally killing that child. The "forced birth" narrative is a desperate reframing of the pro-life argument that turns pregnancy—something beautiful—into an image of incarceration and torture. It is a shameful approach.

Good News, Bad News

The *Dobbs* decision did not produce unalloyed good news. Ideally, the Supreme Court would officially have recognized the humanity and legal personhood of children in the womb and dealt a death blow to the abortion industry. Instead, the justices decided to return the question of abortion to the states.

The good news is that the unhinged individuals making terrible arguments, violently attacking pregnancy help centers, shrieking in the streets as they play-act child killing, are far outnumbered by the millions of people who reside in the "mushy middle." These unpersuaded (but persuadable) individuals are the key targets for pro-life messaging.

We have the message and the means to win them. Most have never heard a comprehensive case for the sanctity of human life; but when they do (as you will read later), many alter their position.

So, take heart. Solutions are coming.

But first, I need to address the greatest challenge in the battle to stop the intentional killing of children in the womb: the exponential expansion in the use of the abortion pill, the most nefarious strategy imaginable. The next chapter covers this major pivot of the abortion industry, which retreated and retrenched in abortion states. Then, by leveraging medical technology that mushroomed during COVID, and building a wall of protection around abortionists, they have expanded farther than any bricks-and-mortar abortion business could have dreamed.

I'll show you how they did it.

CHAPTER 3

Retreat, Retrench, and the Power of the Abortion Pill Pivot

Abortion grows in secret and in silence. For decades, abortion advocates machinated to hide from the public the truth about fetal development and the nature of abortion. The existence of *Roe v. Wade* shielded the abortion industry from meaningful regulation, even though most legal scholars considered it a poorly-decided case. Even liberal Supreme Court Justice Ruth Bader Ginsburg agreed with pro-lifers that the reasoning in *Roe* was flawed. That's a pretty good indication that its proponents were destined to lose.[47]

Planned Parenthood locations shuttered across the country in the wake of the *Dobbs* decision. But the jubilation in pro-life circles was premature.

Rather than acknowledging defeat, Planned Parenthood decided to close shop in hostile territory and regroup in abortion-friendly states. There, funding would continue to flow, abortion facilities would persist unabated, while supportive legislatures would shield abortion operations from outside interstate interference. From this protective high ground, they could use a tiny, insidious methodology to continue their child-killing efforts even in the most staunchly pro-life states in the country.

The abortion pill is the single most successful attack of the abortion industry on states and people who want to outlaw intentional child-killing.

By the end of this chapter, you will see how the abortion industry is hardly in retreat, how abortion pills have become the focused strategy, and why eliminating abortion pills (and, by extension, abortion-pill abortions) is virtually impossible.

Despite these challenges, there is a way forward. Initially it will come through additional protective legislation, but the rest of the answers you will discover in Part Two.

Planned Parenthood: Retreat or Retrenching?

Even before the *Dobbs* decision, pro-life protection laws in states such as Texas were already forcing the closure of abortion facilities. For a long time, Planned Parenthood tried to persuade the American public that abortion was only a small part of what it touted as the much-needed services it provides. It claimed that elective abortion made up just three percent of its overall services.

But if that were true, then why did over half of Planned Parenthood locations close their doors throughout Texas between 2013 and 2014, once understandable restrictions on abortion were advanced in Texas?[48] Wouldn't it still be able to offer the other supposed 97 percent of its services? The action of abortionists revealed, to the surprise of no one, that abortion facilities are in the business of intentional child-killing. When that aspect of their business model was threatened, facilities closed their doors.

In Texas, initially this meant retreating to more favorable territory, such as Houston, where Planned Parenthood had opened one of the nation's largest abortion facilities. With the coming of the *Dobbs* decision, however, Planned Parenthood abandoned even that building and decamped for abortion-favoring states such as New Mexico. Abortion businesses throughout pro-life states were shuttered.

Cue declarations of victory in the pro-life camp. The enemy was in retreat! But were they, really?

'Telehealth,' Shield Laws, and Abortion Pills

If abortionists could not legally set up shop physically in pro-life states, then they would regroup in abortion states. Friendly governors would divert funds to at least partially replace federal money that had become unavailable. Because the COVID era ushered in an explosion of telehealth, abortionists latched on to that technology – and the terminology – as a way to export abortion to states with pro-life protection laws.[49] It didn't matter where the patient lived, so long as the abortionist operated inside the boundaries of an abortion state.

'Telehealth' or 'E-tail Abortions'?

While it is true that some abortionists speak with pregnant women on the phone or via video chat (the "tele" in "telehealth"), that experience is far from universal. In many instances, the ordering of abortion pills takes place entirely online, the woman speaks directly to no one, and the pills are purchased and shipped.

Not only is there often no "tele" in "telehealth" regarding abortion delivery, there certainly is no "health." Pregnancy is not a disease. Preborn children are not tumors. And, as you will see below, not only are chemical abortions deadly to children, they are often harmful to women. So in the interest of truth in terminology, I will refer to this experience as "e-tail abortion." Far from true medical care, e-tail abortion is instead often a commercial transaction similar to the retail purchase of any product online.

Shield Laws as Offensive Weapons Against Pro-Life States

To protect abortionists from criminal, civil, or even insurance-oriented liability, twenty-two states enacted "shield laws" through legislation or executive action. In at least eight states, the shield law explicitly protects abortionists who interact with patients across state lines.[50]

Shield laws have had a devastating effect on pro-life states. E-tail abortions increased approximately 50 percent between 2022 and 2023.

As *Mother Jones* reported: "The increase is partly thanks to the rise of shield laws, which protect providers who virtually prescribe and mail abortion pills to people in states with abortion bans, according to one of the report's co-authors, Ushma Upadhyay, a researcher at the University of California, San Francisco."[51]

Imagine, for a moment, that a state such as Oregon, where physician-assisted suicide is legal, decided to test the limits of shield law protection. What if they included not just their abortionists but their euthanasia doctors under such a law? Imagine the response of states that have rejected physician-assisted suicide to an influx of euthanasia drugs prescribed and shipped to people living in life-affirming states, after just two online interviews with euthanasia-supporting physicians in Oregon. Suddenly, hundreds of people drop dead. The justification for such a shield law for euthanasia enthusiasts is already in place. If a practice is legal in Oregon, then the state will protect *any* physician acting under the laws of Oregon from *any* criminal or civil action brought by people from another state jurisdiction. How would life-affirming states react? What kind of outcry would that produce?

We should be hearing precisely that kind of outcry right now . . . but we're not. While this example is hypothetical, the following story isn't.

A mother in Louisiana contacted New York-based abortionist Dr. Margaret Carpenter online, asking her to provide abortion pills. Carpenter never examined the woman, who was, herself, not pregnant at all. Rather, the woman's daughter was pregnant. It was reported that the daughter felt excited about the pregnancy, evidenced by her planning a gender reveal party.[52] Carpenter shipped the pills and the mother coerced her daughter to take them, intentionally killing the child in her womb.

The girl's mother was arrested—it is against the law in every state to coerce a pregnant woman to have an abortion—but Louisiana District Attorney Tony Clayton didn't stop there. He also indicted Carpenter for "criminal abortion" and is seeking to have her extradited from New York to Louisiana to answer the charge.[53]

As expected, New York Governor Kathy Hochul blocked Carpenter's extradition under New York's "shield laws." Carpenter had been sued the previous year by Texas Attorney General Ken Paxton for a similar violation. Two separate states filed criminal or civil complaints against an abortionist, one issuing an extradition order; but a third state's governor blocked the perpetrator from having to answer the charges.

Such a legal deadlock should invite federal intervention. So far, it hasn't. One wonders whether the hypothetical Oregon euthanasia example above will remain hypothetical for long.

How Abortion Pills Further Abortion Ideology

The proliferation of the abortion pill is a masterstroke by the abortion industry, which pitched the pills using the same rhetoric that surrounded elective surgical abortion from its inception. Abortion pills, women are told, are a legal, effective, and safe method by which to "terminate a pregnancy" in early stages. While the abortion pill had been prescribed for decades before the *Dobbs* decision, in the years leading up to *Dobbs* its use exploded.[54] Depending on which reporting entity you believe, abortion pills currently account for 65-70+ percent of all elective abortions in the United States.

Safe and Effective?

The abortion "pill" protocol in fact requires two types of pills: mifepristone and misoprostol. Together, these drugs are often referred to as a "medication abortion." But "medication" refers to a drug used to treat or cure illnesses, and pregnancy is not an illness. Therefore, I will use the terms "abortion pill" or "chemical abortion" to refer to these two drugs, either together or individually, when used in abortions.

Mifepristone is a progesterone blocker that stops the developing child from receiving nutrients. This makes the womb a hostile environment.

Misoprostol causes the cervix to dilate and the uterus to contract, forcing the child from the womb. The FDA approves the use of the abortion pill through ten weeks of pregnancy.

When pro-abortion circles expressed concern that mifepristone might become a highly-regulated drug, some states began to stockpile it. Washington, for example, purchased 30,000 doses of mifepristone.[55] Apparently, that was unnecessary, as abortion advocates published studies touting the efficacy of "misoprostol-only abortions."[56] Doctors originally developed misoprostol as an ulcer treatment. Under the heading "Important Information," the warning label says, "Do not use this drug if you become pregnant."[57] That caution served as an instruction manual for abortion proponents. The intentional death of a child by induced miscarriage was precisely what they wanted to cause.

Combining the two drugs makes chemical abortions the most "successful." When mifepristone is taken alone, the child has up to a twenty-five percent chance of surviving.[58] Misoprostol-only abortions might result in live births, but at such a young age in her development, the premature child has only a small chance of survival.[59] Louise Adsett, a midwife in Australia testifying before the Queensland legislature, reported, "Just recently a mother decided to abort her baby at nineteen weeks. The same Misoprostol regime was started and this little baby was born alive—again, moving, gasping for air and having a palpable heart rate and, once again, weighed over 400 grams."[60] The child did not survive.

When mifepristone is coupled with misoprostol, the chance for the child's survival is virtually nil. It is hard to imagine a drug protocol labeled as "safe" which results in the death of nearly every child in the womb when administered to the mother.

Serious adverse effects arising from the use of chemical abortion pills are reported as less than .5 percent on the FDA-approved Mifeprex insert. A 2013 study of abortion pill users found that .3 percent of research subjects required hospitalization, while .1 percent required blood transfusion.

Nearly 5 percent of these women had "treatment failure," requiring a subsequent surgical abortion.[61]

But it turns out that the abortion pill isn't as safe for the mother as many initially thought (see the next chapter). Even so, there is a push to extend the use of abortion pills later and later into pregnancy.

Later Term Abortion Pill Usage

The FDA limit on abortion-pill abortions is ten weeks from the last menstrual cycle. But that didn't stop Aid Access, a telemedicine abortion company, from shipping pills to "Briana," even though she reported being "at least five weeks beyond the FDA's 10-week limit."[62] Her story, appearing in the *Washington Post* on April 11, 2024, is harrowing: "She ran to the bathroom, she recalled in interviews and a journal entry, where she felt a mass larger than her palm drop into the toilet."

Notice the language choice. When you read an article on a medical topic and see something described as "a mass," what immediately comes to mind? For most of us, a "mass" means a tumor or cancer. So already in the story, the preborn child is dehumanized and turned into a negative clump of dangerous cells.

But Briana's nightmare had just begun.

Emails from the Aid Access doctors had explained what to expect after taking the abortion pills: "nausea, vomiting, chills, blood clots and a fetus at least the size of an orange." They failed to mention that her child would be attached to her by an umbilical cord. She told the investigator that she stood there for fifteen minutes, wondering whether she should manually pull out the cord. A hotline worker told her what Aid Access had not, that she still had the placenta inside her and she would need to push it out: "When you feel the next contraction, I want you to push like you're giving birth."

No one told Briana that she would give birth that day to a dead, fully-formed child. At the bottom of her toilet bowl, she could see the child's head and long legs. Looking back on the experience, she said, "I felt like a monster."

It may surprise you to learn that Briana's story appeared in an article with a decidedly pro-abortion slant, even though the essay contains more than one story of women traumatized by the abortion pill experience. One, a fifteen-year-old girl, called a hotline when the deceased child she delivered was too large to flush down the toilet. She asked the operator whether her actions made her a bad person. Others are described as "traumatized."

The abortion horror stories revealed in the *Washington Post* essay focus exclusively on the devastating experiences of the women. Readers are expected to conclude that none of this would happen if not for pro-life states banning abortion on demand. To the writer of that article, abortion is nothing more than another form of health care that women need. By refusing to acknowledge the true victims in these narratives—the children in the womb who have been cut off from vital nutrition and then forced out of the womb prematurely to die—the author hides the most important truth: abortion pills intentionally kill children.

Abortion advocates obscure language.
As long as they can keep people believing that abortion is anything other than what it is – intentional child killing – they can prevail. Abortion grows in secret; its ally is silence.
It cannot withstand the truth.

Other recent stories describe late-term chemical abortions. Some of them depict criminal acts, while others are presented as scientific research.

In Nebraska, Jessica Burgess and her daughter, Celeste, conspired together to use abortion pills to intentionally kill Celeste's child. The daughter was twenty-four weeks into her pregnancy, so her actions violated the state's twenty-week limit on abortions. As in the Dr. Carpenter case previously described, Jessica acquired the pills for her daughter. In messages on Facebook, Celeste "talks about how she can't wait to get the 'thing' out of her body,' a detective wrote in court documents. 'I will finally be able to wear jeans,' she says in one of the messages."[63] After delivering her dead child, the mother and daughter burned the body and buried it.

In addition to the popular press, medical journals are reporting research on the effectiveness of later-term chemical abortions at thirteen weeks' gestation and beyond. In *Contraception: X*, researchers in 2021 discussed the use of the abortion pill by pregnant women who were thirteen to fifteen weeks into their pregnancy (though a sizeable percentage of the sample, 22 percent, were sixteen or more weeks pregnant). The researchers concluded that these e-tailed chemical abortions were safe and effective. "Telemedicine or provision for home use of medical abortion at 13 weeks or more gestation appear to be generally safe and acceptable up to 16 weeks' gestation," they reported, but then added, "however, risks of abortion failure and provoking a premature delivery occurred among those with gestational ages greater than 20 weeks, as was decreased acceptability of the method."[64] Premature delivery of a woman's living child was listed as a "risk."

Similarly, a 2024 research article in the same journal surveyed chemical abortion outcomes in women between eighteen weeks and twenty-three weeks and six days of pregnancy. Despite one patient suffering a uterine rupture, the authors note, "Using medication to induce abortion in the second trimester can include expulsion at home, as was true for three patients in this study. Patient counseling and materials should include information on what to expect and how to respond if expulsion happens outside the clinic setting."[65]

In the *Washington Post* story cited earlier, although Briana was fifteen weeks into her pregnancy, her e-tail abortion company failed to advise her about the umbilical cord. She felt horrified when she saw a fully-formed baby in the toilet. But should it surprise us that abortion businesses do not choose to accurately describe, much less show photographs, of what these mothers should expect to see? They seem happy to recommend that women deliver, at home, children even more developed than Briana's.

Blake Zwerling and his abortion-friendly research team from The Society of Family Planning made recommendations in 2025 for abortion pill use from the fourteenth week through the twenty-seventh week of pregnancy. Compare their advice with stories, admittedly rare, of children being born as early as twenty-one weeks and yet growing up to lead normal lives.[66] Children born at twenty-four weeks have nearly a 70 percent chance of survival; and for children born prematurely at twenty-six weeks (still within Zwerling's recommended age range for chemical abortion), nearly 90 percent survive.[67]

Some researchers callously suggest that in cases where the targeted child is "approaching viability" that the abortionist should kill the child first, while he is still in the womb, by injecting his heart with a drug such as digoxin, before beginning the chemical abortion.[68] An essay in the *American Journal of Obstetrics and Gynecology* advised: "Inducing fetal asystole [stopping the child's heart] before medication abortion at near-viable gestational durations to avoid signs of life at time of expulsion is practiced widely for legal considerations as well as patient and provider comfort."[69] The researchers advise killing the child before delivery to avert any potential legal problems resulting from a live baby, when the intent of the procedure is to produce a dead one. The birth of a living, premature child is considered a risky complication, because seeing a squirming child, with a palpable heartbeat and gasping to take a breath, might upset the mother and/or the abortionist.

How Chemical Abortion Affects Worldview Creation

When I train pastors and laypeople about abortion, I always stress that abortion is not primarily a political, moral, or spiritual issue. In fact, abortion is not primarily an *issue* at all. Abortion is an action that produces casualties. Still, abortion as an act perpetrated and shaped by culture certainly does have political, moral, and spiritual implications, all three of which are a part of worldview creation.

Language

While I've devoted a later chapter entirely to language, here I want to point out the effects of the specific word choices employed by the journalists and researchers cited above. Repeatedly, the child in the womb is identified as a "fetus," which would be fine if everyone knew that "fetus" is just a Latin term meaning "little one" or "offspring." Instead, to many people, the word "fetus" represents something other than human, or something that may *become* human but isn't quite yet. I have seen many short videos filmed on college campuses in which students respond to any claim of human worth for children in the womb with screams of "It's a FETUS!" In Nebraska, Celeste described her child as "the thing."

In one story told in the *Washington Post* article, the author describes the trauma of a woman identified as Angel after she "passed a fetus larger than she expected."[70] People "pass" kidney stones, not children.

The essay in the *American Journal of Obstetrics and Gynecology* describes the forced premature birth following a chemical abortion as "expulsion." Typically, "expulsion" occurs when governments remove unwanted aliens living illegally in their jurisdictions, or when schools permanently remove unruly students. Most of us do not associate the word with childbirth. Even the term "stillborn" contains the word "born," not "expelled."

The rhetorical purpose of associating dehumanizing and negative terms with preborn children, and the process of intentionally killing and disposing of them, is to create a worldview that hides the target of abortion and whitewashes the violence inherent in the act.

Desensitization

In 2014, I went to an early screening of the film *The Giver*, based on Lois Lowry's young adult novel. Like many such books and films of the time, the setting featured a dystopian near future when people neither carried, birthed, or cared for their own biological children. The incubated children who did not reach a predetermined weight were euthanized.

One scene involved a child, from a set of twins, who had failed to thrive. The main character's father is a "Nurturer," and ironically it falls to him to kill the weak. He picks up the baby and lethally injects the child while cheerfully speaking to him. Once the drug does its work, he places the baby in a box and pushes it into a chute, like one might do for dirty laundry or garbage. As the child disappears, he says, "Goodbye, little guy" and exits.[71]

I had read the book before seeing the film and was curious about the audience's reaction if that scene were included. Viewers gasped in horror at the cavalier way the adult killed the innocent baby. In that moment, I felt hope for this generation. They had witnessed a fictional horror, which had produced in them a very real and appropriate moral response.

But as the number of at-home chemical abortions continue to rise, I fear that young women will become desensitized to killing. A TikTok video shown at a banquet I keynoted in Chattanooga, Tennessee, opened with a young woman pressing a blister pack of the abortion pill to the screen. She pulls it back, then the scene cuts to her holding mifepristone in one hand and what appears to be an energy drink in the other. She announces, "There will be no birth and I deserve cake!" She takes the pill.

Time passes. She returns to the screen in a different outfit and hairstyle. "Trigger warning," she says, and then counts down: "Three, two, one." She holds a transparent baggie to the screen containing what appears to be her dead child with an umbilical cord attached. The woman looks into the camera and asks, "Does it look like me?" Then she smiles.

Looking closely, you can clearly see the child's head and its arm and leg buds. The child is developmentally a human fetus, so yes, it looks like her. The level of depravity is jarring, all the more so because this woman determined to make her child killing a public act. And then she openly mocked her victim.

For many years, pro-life leaders have argued with good cause that if people really knew and believed that preborn children were morally indistinguishable from toddlers, the knowledge would go a long way toward ending abortion. A common argument used by pro-life advocates, popularized by Life Training Institute's Scott Klusendorf, contends that there is no significant moral distinction between the embryo you used to be and the (toddler, teen, adult) you are now that would have justified killing you then, but not now.

But a new cultural wave is attempting to turn that argument on its head. The response goes something like this: "You're right, there is no significant moral distinction. We think it would have been okay to kill you then, and so we'd have no qualms about killing you now."

Initiation into the Tribe

One of the most nefarious outcomes of the shift to abortion pills is what it does to the women taking them. Not long ago, a woman with a friend in the car might have driven past an old building, teared up, pointed, and sobbed, "That is where that doctor did that to me!" There was a dedicated building, staffed by professional abortionists, who took the woman's money, sedated her, and then killed and removed her child from her body. It happened "there" and it was done by "them."

But the abortion pill has changed all of that. It reminds me of what happened with the pornography industry.

When I was a kid in the 1960s, about the only way I would happen upon an image of a naked woman was if a friend's dad or brother had a secret stash of *Playboys*, or if, while I was out playing in the woods, I stumbled over some torn-out pages from a "skin magazine." Back then, for a man to watch an actual pornographic film often required driving to a seedy part of town and risking that some acquaintance might witness him buying a ticket and entering the X-rated theater. Later, when such films became available in the back room of a video rental store, a patron still had to interact with sales staff and might risk being seen at the store by friends. Significant peer pressure existed to *not* do that.

Then streaming arrived. Now, in the privacy of a bathroom, dorm room, bedroom or home, people may watch footage more debauched than virtually anything their grandparents could have imagined. Over time, usage became normalized. Today, college students and others openly admit to watching porn. It's so bad that when the Barna research group surveyed clergy, 21 percent of youth pastors and 11 percent of other pastors admitted that they were currently struggling with watching porn.[72] When pornography watching became private, it massively increased the population of watchers even as it normalized the behavior. The thinking goes: "if everyone is doing it, can it really be all that bad?"

In much the same way that streaming services privatized porn, the abortion pill – received by mail after an e-tail abortion appointment on a cell phone or online – privatized abortion. No need to risk being seen going into an abortion facility. No need to be accompanied by someone else to get a ride home. The pills come in an unmarked envelope, are consumed in private, and then the dead child frequently splashes into a toilet, where all the evidence that one was ever pregnant gets flushed into the sewer system.

The abortion takes place in the woman's dorm room, bathroom, or bedroom. No impersonal office building or nefarious person exists to point at. The woman has become her own abortionist. She might not have completely known what she was doing or what the outcome would look like, but she does know that she willingly took those pills. Her connection to her abortion is much closer and more personal than it would have been in the past. For many women, it may be a psychological, moral, and spiritual bridge too far to agree that what has occurred in a chemical abortion is the intentional killing of her own child.

For those mothers in anguish or denial, an entire tribe waits to embrace women who abort their children, calling them "brave," a "girl boss," someone expressing her own "bodily autonomy." It's easy to enter such a tribe; initiation is just an action, a story, or a supportive comment away. But it is very difficult to leave.

Watch abortion advocates confront pro-life apologists (particularly women who regret their abortions) on a college campus and you will immediately see what I mean. Angry outbursts, accusations of misogyny, tables flipped, signs destroyed, people cursing those trying to protect the preborn and wishing that the apologist's children were raped. None of these are uncommon occurrences and they happen on college campuses where free speech and open inquiry are supposed to rule the day. Pro-abortion ideology exerts strong peer pressure to conform. Any effort to undermine that narrative is a target, even if the purpose is to help a woman who has changed her mind about abortion.

The Attack on Abortion Pill Reversal

As pregnancy help centers and clinics began offering bioidentical progesterone therapies to women who wanted to save the lives of their children after regretting taking mifepristone, the abortion industry and their state political allies went on the attack.

First up was Colorado; in 2023 its legislature passed a bill that outlawed the use of Abortion Pill Reversal, identifying its use with "unprofessional conduct, effectively outlawing it in Colorado and subjecting providers to professional discipline."[73] Not far behind was California. In September 2023, California Attorney General Rob Bonta sued Heartbeat International and several California-based pregnancy centers, arguing that Abortion Pill Reversal violated California's False Advertising Law and Unfair Competition Law and that it was illegal to offer it to patients as a valid and successful method.[74]

Then in 2024, New York's Attorney General Letitia James also filed suit against Heartbeat International and New York pregnancy centers. She made claims similar to those advanced in California.[75] These states don't want those children to be saved. In fact, the current level of abortion isn't enough, they want more.

Advertising Child Killing in Pro-Life States

Shortly after the *Dobbs* decision, California designated itself an abortion sanctuary state. The California Future of Abortion Council lobbied for, and got, a $200M line item in the state budget to "expand abortion access."[76] California Governor Gavin Newsom, flush with money from his successful reelection campaign, took some of it and placed pro-abortion billboards in seven pro-life states: Texas, Ohio, South Carolina, Indiana, Oklahoma, South Dakota, and Mississippi.[77] In Austin, Texas, the billboard read: "Need an Abortion? California is Ready to Help." At the bottom, he included a scripture verse from Mark 12:31: "Love your neighbor as yourself. There is no greater commandment than these."[78]

The abortion industry in California felt dissatisfied with operating solely within a friendly state. It has a "missionary mindset," desiring to evangelize outside of its safe haven. That means infiltrating states trying to protect the lives of children from those hellbent on killing them. Using a strategy straight from the devil—twisting Scripture to suit their own ends—they cite out of context a verse from the Gospels to make it appear as if intentionally killing children in the womb is an act of loving your neighbor. This, even though *all* children are, just as their mothers and fathers are, made in the image of God, who desires them to be loved and cherished, not killed.

California was hardly alone and billboards aren't the only strategy. Planned Parenthood, leveraging the reach and anonymity of the Internet, in 2019 launched Roo, a chatbot aimed at teenagers.[79] Roo, as you might recall, is also the name of the rambunctious offspring of Kanga in the Winnie the Pooh stories. While writing this paragraph, I logged into the chatbot, identifying myself as a seventeen-year-old girl, a minor. And within a couple of clicks, I was on a page to make an e-tail appointment to get abortion pills.

PlanCPills and Aid Access are websites that guide people to e-tail abortion providers and chemical abortions. The PlanCPills site, for example, forwards curious visitors to Reprolegal, a site that discusses the legal implications of abortion in various states. A visitor who clicks on Tennessee would discover that Tennessee bans abortion and that it is a crime to mail or give abortion pills to a pregnant woman.[80] The page then advises women that they can't be criminally charged for "self-managed" abortions in Tennessee.

Despite explaining that it is illegal to mail or give abortion pills to a pregnant woman in Tennessee, the site links to ineedana.com (as in "I need an abortion") which notes on its landing page: "Need an abortion? No matter what state you live in, you still have options."[81] Filling out the form as a seventeen-year-old, a warning came up saying I would need a notarized consent form from a parent if I wanted to get an abortion out of state. But below that warning appeared options to contact abortion pill providers, with language indicating that even if you lived in a pro-life state, the dispensing state's "shield law" would enable the provider to send the pills. The site notes that legal trouble might await on the receiving end; but as you will discover in chapter ten, the odds are very small that the recipient will be discovered, much less successfully prosecuted. And "just in case," ineedana provides links to a legal hotline. Need to budget? No problem. Ineedana provides an abortion estimate calculator.[82]

Aid Access founder, Dutch physician Rebecca Gomperts, explained in an interview why mail is the perfect workaround:

> In the U.S., there's very strong protection of mail. Even if they track it down, there's no way to prove that anybody took the pills. And to buy the medicines is not against any law. It's not against any

> regulation to get medicines for your own use... Aid Access is about providing information so that people know what their rights are. It's a human right to get abortion pills. Also, if they need to go to the hospital, they can say that they had a miscarriage. It's the same treatment as when you have a medical abortion. And it's nobody's business whether you took the pills or not. What kind of medical care you get doesn't depend on that.[83]

The strategy is all about plausible deniability. And so far, it's working.

Since billboards and websites are expensive to put up and maintain, some abortion providers take a decidedly low-tech, everything-but-the-kitchen-sink, guerilla approach to undermining the laws in pro-life states. Mayday Health, an e-tail abortion information clearinghouse, placed placard ads on top of gasoline pumps in pro-life West Virginia, eastern Kentucky, and Texas which read: "Pregnant? Don't Want to Be?"[84] It went on to use billboard trucks in Tennessee and Iowa, floating billboards in Florida, it flew an ad over the Indianapolis 500 for three days, and published print ads in the hometown papers of the Supreme Court justices that overturned *Roe* in the *Dobbs* decision.[85]

Mayday Health founders argue that they are just spreading information and therefore their activities are protected by the First Amendment. But imagine one of the counties in Nevada where prostitution is legal taking out billboard space near a Mississippi community college inviting young men to lose their virginity at one of their brothels (Nevada outlaws *in-state* advertising for prostitution anywhere outside of the counties where it is legal), or an ad in *The Marine Corps Times* offering sex services to lonely Marines at Camp Pendleton (the Uniform Code of Military Justice makes prostitution a court martial offense). The key question has not been fully litigated. Do states have, or should they have, the right to limit the speech of those who want to use it to encourage, entice, or promote behavior that is legally criminal in that state?

It's Not All Bad News

In this chapter, I've labored to show you how the abortion industry has pivoted since *Dobbs* and how its new strategies have expanded child-killing across the entire U.S. But, in the next chapter, you'll see some of the victories pro-life advocates achieved in the same period. I'll also begin laying the groundwork for current and future efforts required to win this battle for life.

CHAPTER 4

Shining Light on 'E-tail' Abortion

It was a masterstroke. The abortion industry was now expanding abortion into areas of the country that never even knew the shadow of an abortion facility. E-tail abortion – marshalling the power of internet commerce to arrange delivery of chemical abortion pills – brought child-killing technology to every mailbox in America. Shield laws completed the trifecta. It seems like the perfect pivot. But is it?

Weaknesses in the strategy of abortion advocates have begun to show. In this chapter, I want to start by revealing what happens when children in the womb are considered disposable, because that is what abortion teaches those who tolerate it. Then, I'll expose the lies behind abortion pill distribution, and the attacks leveled against the only effective remedy once mothers begin a chemical abortion. Finally, I want to encourage you. There is hope on the horizon for states that want to limit the ability of the abortion industry to target their citizens.

What Happens When a Nation Devalues Life?

In the last chapter I told you the horrifying story of Jessica, a Nebraska woman who conspired with her daughter, Celeste, to use abortion pills to kill Celeste's preborn child. Jessica was prosecuted for her actions and sentenced to two years in prison after she was convicted of illegal abortion and "tampering with human remains." Celeste was sentenced only to ninety days for her role in burning and burying her child's body.[86]

Philosopher Gary M. Atkinson explained in the *International Philosophical Quarterly*, way back in 1974, that arguments made in support of abortion on demand, if accepted, would also support infanticide and involuntary euthanasia. It starts this way: "Acceptance is first gained for abortion by emphasizing irrelevant or even imaginary distinctions between the fetus and the newborn child. For example, one speaks of 'fetal tissue' or 'developing human tissue' or 'the products of pregnancy' while refusing to allow as linguistically proper any reference to the fetus as a child."[87]

But the child in the womb *is* a living human person, regardless of the language used to describe her. If you doubt that, compare the dehumanizing language abortion supporters use against the way parents talk about their wanted children throughout the pregnancy. Many celebrities have little difficulty recognizing the humanity of their wanted children in the womb. Hilaria Baldwin, wife of actor Alec Baldwin, posted a sonogram image of their developing baby in 2022. *The Daily Mail* article describes the child as a baby girl and as her "daughter." Hilaria captioned the ultrasound photo: "There she is!!!"[88] Actress Kate Mara, announcing her coming baby with husband Jamie Bell, shared a photo of what appeared to be the couple walking together, captioning it "There are three of us in this pic."[89] Three what? Three people. Three of "us."

Not Every Culture Values Human Life

I occasionally remind myself that many ancient civilizations had no problem with sacrificing children or adults when they felt it would help them solve spiritual, political, or territorial issues. These same cultures also had no reservations about enslaving other human beings.

You might like to believe that all people at all times have always agreed that human lives are inherently valuable. But you'd be wrong.

As Tom Holland points out in *Dominion: How the Christian Revolution Remade the World*, the idea that individual human lives have significant worth is both fairly recent and localized. For most of human history, and in most of the world, human life was *not* treasured. The value of human life is grounded firmly in the Christian idea of the image-bearer. What happens when people believe no God exists whose image they bear? Once they embrace the idea that humans are no more worthy of respect than any other animal, they cease to believe that any moral values exist to which all humans are beholden. And in those cultures, human life becomes both cheap and disposable.

Americans are rapidly moving toward (if we haven't already reached) the kind of world Paul warns of in Romans 1, when people "exchanged the truth of God for a lie, and worshiped and served the creature rather than the Creator, who is blessed forever. Amen."[90] When civilizations abandon transcendent truth, only transcendent lies exist to replace them. Where no law exists, lawlessness abounds. Where there is no shame, people act shamefully. No culture and no nation that openly celebrates despising and slaughtering its own children can long endure.

Not only does abortion show disdain for children in the womb, but the abortion industry is disingenuous about its "care" for pregnant women. And it begins with the common – yet insane – assertion of abortionists that abortion is "safe." You know it's not "safe" for the children it annihilates. Turns out, it's not safe for their mothers, either.

How Safe is the Abortion Pill, Really?

A 2025 study surveying data from insurance providers examining prescriptions and outcomes for nearly 700,000 women spoke volumes regarding the "safety" of taking the abortion pill. As you might expect, women who swallow the abortion industry's claims may be putting themselves at far more risk than they've been led to believe.

Researchers Ryan Anderson and Jamie Bryan Hall from the Ethics and Public Policy Center discovered that the actual level of serious adverse reactions to taking the abortion pill was nearly 11 percent, about twenty-two times higher than the .5 percent adverse reaction rate claimed by the FDA. The adverse reactions they uncovered included incidents "such as emergency room visits, hemorrhage, sepsis, infection, and/or follow-up surgeries for the women who had downed the abortion drug within the last forty-five days."[91]

The effectiveness of APR is what drives the vehemence of its opponents. The last thing they want is a live child, whose very rescue is an indictment of their deadly intent.

Abortion pills sent through the mail to women who have not been examined by a physician carry an additional risk: ectopic pregnancy. Not all children implant in their mother's uterus. Some implant outside, and of these, the overwhelming majority implant in their mother's fallopian tubes. Chemical abortion will not terminate an ectopic pregnancy. But the symptoms of an ectopic pregnancy—vaginal bleeding, abdominal pain, nausea, and fatigue—mimic what women are told to expect during a chemical abortion. As a result, women who use e-tail abortion may think they have completed the procedure, when in fact the child continues to develop. If the fallopian tube ruptures, it places the woman's life at risk.

Dr. Patricia Santiago-Muñoz, an OB/GYN at the University of Texas Southwestern Medical Center, explains, "Though ectopic pregnancies comprise just 1% to 2% of all pregnancies, the condition is the leading cause of pregnancy-related maternal death in the first trimester, usually due to lack of medical intervention."[92]

By August of 2025, twenty-two state attorneys general have requested that the initial safety protocols for the abortion pill, issued in 2000, be reinstated, including limiting the gestational age of the targeted child to seven weeks, requiring the reporting of non-fatal adverse events, and to disallow the mailing of the drugs. But as of the time of this writing, none of these recommendations have been enacted.

Attacking Abortion Pill Reversal

Once women begin surgical abortions, there is virtually no chance to save the life of the child in the womb. Even if the woman regrets her decision to abort her child, the moment of rescue has passed; the child is dead.

Chemical abortions, on the other hand, provide an opportunity that surgical abortions do not. The abortion pill protocol recommended by the FDA advises the pregnant woman to take mifepristone and then wait twenty-four to forty-eight hours before taking misoprostol. Some women feel anxiety and guilt after taking mifepristone, wishing they had a way to undo what they started. Fortunately, there is such a way: bioidentical progesterone.

Mifepristone is a progesterone antagonist; it blocks the ability of progesterone (a naturally-occurring hormone) to prepare a uterine lining so that it may provide the nutrition the newly implanted embryonic child requires. Research shows that women who have taken mifepristone, but who haven't yet taken misoprostol, have a window of time in which to reverse the effects of the first drug. If those women are given bioidentical progesterone (often popularly referred to as Abortion Pill Reversal), they significantly improve their odds of carrying a healthy child.

Women have successfully used oral progesterone for decades to help support their pregnancies. When used under medical supervision the drug is considered safe. You would never know that, however, if you listened to legislators and the Attorneys General in states such as Colorado, California, and New York. As noted in the previous chapter, Colorado passed a bill in 2023 that outlawed the use of Abortion Pill Reversal. Later that year, California sued to prevent the use of Abortion Pill Reversal, arguing that it violated the state's False Advertising Law and Unfair Competition Law. And the following year, New York filed a similar suit making similar claims.

Such legislation and lawsuits might lead uninformed citizens to think that using bioidentical progesteroneas a medical strategy to stop the fatal effects of mifepristone was ineffective at best and dangerous at worst. Opponents claimed there was no evidence to support its successful use. But that claim was both disingenuous and false.

Some Clinical Studies Would Be Immoral

To begin with, getting a true scientific experiment on abortion pill reversal would be a highly immoral pursuit. Imagine inviting to a study one hundred pregnant women, all of whom had taken mifepristone but who now wanted to keep their babies. Since true scientific research requires a control group, only half of the women would be given progesterone while the other half would be given a placebo, dooming nearly half of the children in the womb to a potentially avoidable death. Who would agree to such a trial?

Progesterone is Safe and Effective

Second, research *does* exist supporting the safety and effectiveness of progesterone as a way of overcoming the child-killing propensities of mifepristone. In 2023, *The Linacre Quarterly* published a scoping review (a type of research synthesis that maps existing literature on a broad topic to identify key concepts, research gaps, and types of evidence) conducted by Paul DeBeasi.[93] His findings were astounding. Among women who received progesterone within seventy-two hours of ingesting mifepristone, between 65-69 percent of them (depending on whether the progesterone was injected or taken orally) continued their pregnancy. When women take only mifepristone, do not go on to take misoprostol, and no progesterone is given, the continuing pregnancy rate is 25 percent or less. So, taking bioidentical progesteroneresulted in a success rate more than 176 percent higher than doing nothing. Regarding risk, the review concluded: "There is no increased maternal or fetal risk from using bioidentical progesterone in early pregnancy."[94]

A year later, the *Journal of Obstetrics and Gynaecology Research* published a small pilot study involving only six enrolled subjects. All the women had ingested mifepristone between 5.7 and seventy-two hours before progesterone treatment began. Each woman then received 400 mg of progesterone twice a day for three days, followed by 400 mg of progesterone nightly for the following sixteen days. The result was that one woman miscarried, but five women had "ongoing, live pregnancies" two weeks after the start of the progesterone treatment.[95] Because of the small size of the study, the conclusions were guarded: "Larger clinical trials are required to determine the clinical effectiveness of progesterone-after-mifepristone and, more importantly, how best to serve the health needs of women who decide not to continue with a medical abortion."[96]

APR Court Victories

Despite the legal attacks, the news for centers and clinics offering Abortion Pill Reversal has been promising. And those legal attacks, so far at least, have not succeeded.

In August 2025, United States District Judge Daniel Domenico for the District of Colorado issued a permanent injunction against Colorado's anti-Abortion Pill Reversal law. The following January, Colorado settled a lawsuit with Bella Health (a pregnancy help clinic), with the state paying out over $6 million.[97]

In New York, a district court issued and the Second Circuit Court affirmed a preliminary injunction against Attorney General Letitia James, arguing that her case was unlikely to survive First Amendment scrutiny.[98] In October 2025, a California lawsuit filed against Attorney General Bonta was argued on appeal before the U.S. Court of Appeals for the Ninth Circuit.[99] While the decision is forthcoming at the time I write, the result of the similar lawsuit in New York, coupled with the successful litigation against Colorado's repressive anti-Abortion Pill Reversal legislation, should provide relief.

Based on the track record of abortion states, however, I sincerely doubt this is the last attack that pregnancy centers and clinics will have to endure. In the meantime, e-tail abortion providers continue devising ways to further infiltrate pro-life states—but even there, pro-life states have taken action.

Can Advertising Subvert State Law?

Remember Mayday Health, the group that employed subversive advertising tactics to promote abortion services in South Dakota, a pro-life state? South Dakota sued Mayday Health over its advertising, prompting Mayday to countersue South Dakota in federal court for violating Mayday's First Amendment rights.[100]

In March 2026, South Dakota and Mayday Health reached an agreement, dropping all litigation. Mayday Health agreed to remove all its gas station advertising and promised to cease its pro-abortion campaign.

South Dakota Attorney General Marty Jackley declared victory: "My position has been clear and unwavering, South Dakota law governs, and the misleading advertisements must be, and are, stopped."[101]

Because the South Dakota case was settled, no definitive legal outcome resulted from the dispute. How similar cases get decided will significantly alter the battle lines of abortion advocacy. But this outcome certainly gives us hope.

What Lies Ahead

After the *Dobbs* decision dropped, too many of those who align themselves with the pro-life movement had a momentary feeling that victory had been achieved. *Roe v. Wade* was overturned. Some thought abortion had become illegal. It hadn't been, but such individuals saw only what they wanted to see. The following years have clarified the situation for those watching the redrawing of battle lines.

Far from being decisively defeated, the abortion industry looked soberly at its new condition, assessed strategies, tactics, and developed new approaches. It then retrenched and immediately began marching forward. Unfortunately, the outlook for abortion wasn't nearly as bleak as its unhinged advocates publicly professed.

Post-*Roe*, many observers expected the number of abortions to decrease; they did not. In fact, they increased. By ramping up the abortion pill, concentrating resources in friendly states, and utilizing e-tail and shield laws, the abortion industry has made a mockery of many of the gains pro-life states made right before and after *Dobbs*.

But don't stop reading here! If you do, you might think the outlook for the lives of children in the womb in the United States and beyond appears bleak. It really doesn't. So take heart.

At the beginning of this book, I expressed frustration at authors who spend 98 percent of their pages discussing how our culture, nation, or world got into a particular mess, and only two percent providing what often are imprecise or meager solutions. The situation reminds me of what Melvin Udall (Jack Nicholson) complained to Simon Bishop (Greg Kinnear) in *As Good As It Gets*: "I'm drowning here, and you're describing the water!"[102]

By now, you should have a sufficient grasp of the water threatening to drown us. This book is not a lament, but a call to action—specific, meaningful action. Part Two suggests potent tactics we can employ, from the way we speak to the way we educate, legislate, organize, and move forward. In other words, I'll describe the pivots required to bring a lasting defeat to the evil of abortion.

I wish I could describe "one weird trick" out there that, if employed, would finish the job. It doesn't exist. But in the following pages, you will discover marching orders. Not every chapter will have your name on it. But I have little doubt that if you read with a pen in hand (or a highlighter, or a bookmark), you will discover some concrete tactic you can employ *right now*. Whenever you find an action you can take, flag that page; and as soon as you have finished, go back and determine to implement one or more of those actions.

Perhaps you will find other strategies that require further equipping or organizing. I often tell my audiences, "the obligations that follow from learning the truth about abortion are *your* obligations, and I don't use 'you' in the plural sense." When I say "you," I have in mind every individual who has learned the truth.

If you will prayerfully seek, engage in, and fulfill the obligations within your reach, or even those that currently remain just beyond it, together we can win the fight for life, overwhelmingly. The question is this:

Do you have eyes to see and a willingness to sacrifice something of yourself to save the lives of your littlest neighbors? Let's find out.

PART TWO

THE FIVE STRATEGIC PIVOTS

PIVOT 1

STOP USING THE ABORTION INDUSTRY'S LANGUAGE; ADVANCE YOUR OWN

CHAPTER 5

Clarifying Controversies Requires Concrete Terms

"What, exactly, is child sex trafficking?" I ask a lot of people this question these days. Initially, they look at me quizzically, as if to say, "Um, what part of that don't you understand?"

Undaunted, I press forward. "It's not a trick question," I reply. "What is child sex trafficking?" Respondents shrug, then say, "Well, it's when children are trafficked or sold for sex." When I ask whether that would be wrong, or if their church would have any problem preaching against child sex trafficking, they think I have lost my mind. But I haven't.

I'm making a point.

No one has to wonder what's at stake in child sex trafficking. The phrase tells you everything you need to know. The revulsion people feel when they hear that term is both justifiably intense and instantaneous. No one needs to parse the language or engage in nuance based on the rationale offered by child sex traffickers. Everybody knows that child sex trafficking is wrong; except, I would imagine, sex traffickers, who see it as nothing more than a form of property management and rental income.

The term "child sex trafficking" is clear, unlike the term "abortion." Just listen to the divergent ways people talk about abortion. Its advocates often use code words such as "choice," "reproductive justice" or "reproductive freedom" to cloud the nature of what abortion truly is. If you were to choose language to describe "elective abortion" with the same degree of precision used in naming "child sex trafficking," then it could very accurately be described as "intentional child killing."

Imagine what might happen if citizens began to speak openly about intentional child killing. Would any amount of intentional child killing be deemed acceptable? Would people advocate in our public spaces for certain exceptions to a total ban on intentional child killing? Can you imagine someone creating billboards trying to sell the public on the idea that intentional child killing is fine, so long as only the very youngest children are killed? I don't imagine that you can.

Am I now engaging in some form of gross exaggeration? Am I guilty of fearmongering or using unjustifiable emotional appeals to try to win the point?

When defining terms, it is crucial that each word in the term, as well as the term as a whole, reflects reality. Otherwise, you can fall into what I call the "hot dog" fallacy. You can define "hot" using specific temperature ranges and define "dog" as a canine, but if you put those two words together—"hot dog"—you probably won't be interested in eating the result.

I will start this chapter by breaking down the term "intentional child killing" to show that in each of its parts and as a whole, it is a clearer, more descriptive term for the act currently referred to as "elective abortion."

Abortion is Intentional Child Killing

All disciplines use technical terms as a kind of shorthand that their members immediately apprehend, but which can sound obscure to those on the outside. Nothing is inherently wrong with this practice. Using technical language makes it easier and quicker for people inside a discipline to communicate with each other. But it does set up a "terminology wall" between those on the inside and those on the outside—and the lack of transparency can lead people to wrong conclusions.

Since the act of abortion takes place primarily inside the medical community, abortionists and their advocates cloak themselves in the language of medicine. In the modern West, medicine is a branch of science and as such enjoys all the privileges associated with being the most widely-accepted way of knowing. Let me show you how abortion advocates exploit that advantage.

Abortion advocates manage the idea of "unborn" or "preborn" children simply by acting as if they don't exist. Instead, they prefer euphemisms such as "pregnancy tissue" or "the uterine contents." Instead of using the term that most individuals, including Planned Parenthood, have historically used for preborn children, "baby," the abortion industry insists on using what it calls "medically accurate" terms such as "zygote," "embryo," "fetus," and "neonate." (Note that *none* of these terms undermine the fact that preborn children are human persons. The terms simply employ technical language for certain stages of that human's development.)

Concepts frame reality. In the womb of a pregnant woman resides her child. Any argument that denies the mother/child relationship is crafted solely to break that parental bond. It is a lie, and must, therefore, be vigorously opposed.

Why use these terms? It's not to increase the understanding of those hearing them. Rather, they're employed to achieve a persuasive objective. Abortion advocates never want it to enter your mind that a real, live, distinct, whole, innocent human being is being intentionally and physically destroyed by the act of abortion. They know from experience that many individuals don't think of an "embryo" or a "fetus" as a human being. Watch public exchanges between pro-life advocates and abortion supporters (videos on TikTok and Facebook Reels abound) and you will quickly see how abortion advocates use these tactics.

More than half a century ago, Gary M. Atkinson predicted this strategy of abortion advocates. They intend to prohibit the use of the term "baby" in order to create a mental and moral chasm between what the word "child" represents on one side (including the inescapable connection to her mother) and what abortion-industry approved terms such as "products of pregnancy" or "fetal tissue" represent on the other (mere biological products with no relational connections).[103] By changing the way people think, by replacing children with things, abortion advocates paved the way for abortion on demand, as well as for the introduction of infanticide and involuntary euthanasia.

If protectors of children in the womb have any hope of reestablishing the moral, intellectual, and parental connection between the being inside the womb and the mother and father who created her, they need to look at a new term for discussing elective abortion. Intentional child killing is that term.

The Act is Intentional Killing

It seems silly that I should need to define "intentional killing." An intentional killing occurs whenever someone purposefully takes the life of something living. Intentional killing comes in many forms: hit men, people who commit crimes of passion, or armed citizens engaging in acts of self-defense, for example. Not all intentional killing is wrong or even punishable.

When soldiers engage in combat or when people act in defense of themselves or other innocent persons, they don't face arrest or imprisonment. What often determines the moral or legal dimension of intentional killing is the target. When hit men kill selected innocent strangers for money, that action is clearly illegal. When a home invader threatens to rape and kill a woman at knifepoint and she responds by shooting him with a pistol, that action is self-defense and the woman likely will not be prosecuted.

Abortion's own practitioners, many of whom are licensed medical doctors, do not deny that abortion is intentional killing. The child in the womb, from the moment of his or her conception, is certainly alive. David

Boonin, in *A Defense of Abortion*, makes it clear that he understands that the "little boy at an early stage in his physical development" (which Boonin identifies as the potential target for elective abortion) is, in fact, the same little boy he has photos of on his desk, playing in the grass, enjoying the beach.[104] Boonin simply argues that the little boy in the womb, his son, is too young to count as a human person deserving of protection from those who wish to intentionally kill him. Boonin explicitly writes that it would be "morally permissible to end his life at this point." Boonin, and other defenders of abortion, know that abortion represents intentional killing.

Planned Parenthood's pre-1963 brochure *Plan Your Children for Health and Happiness* admitted that "abortion kills the life of a baby after it has begun."[105] Mary Elizabeth Williams describes the preborn child as "a life worth sacrificing."[106] Abortion-rights advocate Camille Paglia openly admits that "abortion is murder, the extermination of the powerless by the powerful." Abortionist Warren Hern, a notorious late-term abortionist, and Billie Corrigan explain:

> We have reached a point in this particular technology [late-term abortion] where there is no possibility of denying an act of destruction. It is before one's eyes. The sensations of dismemberment flow through the forceps like an electric current. It is the crucible of a raging controversy, the confrontation of a modern existential dilemma. The more we seem to solve the problem, the more intractable it becomes.[107]

In the study they published, Hern and Corrigan admit that some of their own surgical assistants "described dreams they had related to D & E [dilation and evacuation, an abortion technique often used for late-term abortion]. Both described dreams of vomiting fetuses along with a sense of horror. Other dreams fixated on the need to protect others from viewing fetal parts.[108] Such responses are consistent with the types of incidents suffered by individuals experiencing traumatic stress.

For those willing to continue performing late-term abortions, the feeling subsided over time. People can get used to just about anything. But it is telling that "some staff members are unable to assist with late abortion because of their reaction to it.... Reactions to the fetus ranged from purposefully not looking at it, to shock, dismay, amazement, disgust, fear, and sadness."[109] Hardly the responses one would expect from people merely removing "pregnancy tissue" or engaging in "fundamental health care."

But they describe precisely the emotional trauma one would anticipate among those who have participated in the intentional killing of a child.

The Target is the Child

Most discussions about abortion focus on the developmental stage of the preborn human being. The argument about developmental stages and the inadequacy of development as a rationale to make abortion morally permissible has often been discussed (see my earlier book, *Contenders*; Scott Klusendorf's *The Case for Life*; Christopher Kaczor's *The Ethics of Abortion*; and innumerable other books and articles). I will not repeat that analysis here. But it is important to demonstrate that degree of development is a terrible standard for determining who counts as a person. Relying on gestational age centers biology as the main point, often ignoring how familial relationships are key to the discussion surrounding abortion.

Kimberly Ells, policy advisor for Family Watch International, perfectly paints the natural, biological connection between children and parents:

> The story of every person's life begins at this same place: mother, baby, and a cord connecting the two. And somewhere—often right there looking on—is a father. The father is the second person to whom the baby belongs and on whom the child has an unquestionable claim. Unless the eggs of one woman have been transferred to the womb of another, the child who emerges from a woman's womb is her biological child, bearing her genetic material and formed from her own body. This tethering of a child to mother and mother to child

> ensures that every baby ever born is known and, usually, claimed by at least one person: its mother. No one is born without being tethered to a specific person, and that person is always a woman.[110]

Abortion advocates are so determined to ignore this connection that they sometimes fail to mention it, even to the women whose children they are helping to abort. I've already mentioned a *Washington Post* story, describing the horrifying experience of Briana, a thirty-four-year-old Alabama woman.[111] Briana was tethered—not to pregnancy tissue, not to the products of conception, not to her uterine contents—but to her child. The umbilical cord provided a grim reminder that drove home the fact that she had intentionally killed the child she had, for a time, nourished through that connection.

The Lure of 'Freedom'

The goal of abortion advocacy is not solely to "terminate a pregnancy" (all pregnancies, because they are temporary conditions and not "things," terminate, generally around forty weeks), but to kill a child. As noted in chapter one, former Secretary of Transportation, Pete Buttigieg, openly discussed the "benefits" of abortion. He noted that the "advantages" of abortion are not limited to women but included "freedom" for men.[112]

Abortion, however, does not unburden a man from pregnancy. Despite contemporary claims to the contrary, it is biologically impossible for men to become pregnant. So, what kind of freedom does abortion grant to men who impregnate women? Freedom from the continued existence of their own children. Freedom from parenting, even from the financial obligations associated with caring for one's own children. Some men sadly abandon their children, while others work with a cooperative mother to place the children they created with another family through adoption. Both acts "free" a man from the perceived financial burden of parenting. The only unique "freedom" abortion provides to the father is freedom from the emotional, psychological, financial, or parental obligations of a live child . . . *his* child.

The Right to No Living Offspring

To demonstrate that the aim of elective abortion is not merely the "termination of a pregnancy" but the elimination of the man and woman's offspring, just look to the futurist literature about artificial wombs. The purpose of the technology is purportedly to solve problems, such as ectopic pregnancy. Currently, we have no viable way to take a child embedded outside the uterus (a child growing in her mother's fallopian tube, for example) and successfully transfer her into her mother's womb, regardless of how "wanted" that child might be. Treatment for ectopic pregnancies, therefore, which directly threaten the life of the mother, require the removal of the child in her embryonic developmental state. Unfortunately, such children have not sufficiently developed to survive outside the womb. We do not yet possess the technology to save such children's lives.

But the current state of medical technology has not stopped cultural analysts and moral philosophers from considering whether the successful, future development of artificial wombs might undermine the case for elective abortion. The existence of an artificial womb would eliminate the physical burden of pregnancy on the body of the woman. It would "terminate her pregnancy" without destroying the child. Would this provide a win-win scenario for everyone? Philosopher Christopher Kaczor, writing in 2005, held out hope that artificial wombs might end the abortion debate:

> ...the vast majority of defenders of abortion who have written about the topic in scholarly journals and books do not defend a right of extermination but rather the right of extraction. The termination of pregnancy, and not the termination of human life, is their stated goal. If they are consistent with what they have written, it would seem that the vast majority of these people could accept the use of artificial wombs in lieu of abortion.[113]

But a brief look at the arguments advanced by abortion advocates reveals plainly that terminating a pregnancy, without also annihilating the child, misses one inherent goal of elective abortion. Rosalind Moran and Julie Zhao explain that at least one aim of abortion, even if artificial wombs were available to gestate the child, is to make sure one has no living children:

> The reality is that some women who choose abortion do so not only to end the pregnancy—preserving bodily autonomy—but also to avoid becoming a biological mother. Ectogenesis would still make her a biological mother against her will, and using it as an alternative to traditional abortion could therefore violate her reproductive autonomy.[114]

The writers note that the potential social stigma and emotional guilt a mother might feel from choosing to use an artificial womb (and, it is implied, placing the child for adoption) should outweigh the right of the woman's child to remain alive.

Beyond Birth

Even in the present state of technology, such arguments have been used to justify abortion over adoption. Additionally, imagine if such arguments were extended to children already in incubators, which perform many of the functions of an artificial womb for children of a more advanced gestational age.

In the minds of some, even live birth does not eliminate the possibility of "freedom from offspring." The title of Alberto Giubilini and Francesca Minerva's essay "After-Birth Abortion: Why Should the Baby Live?" creates a euphemism for infanticide and then unpacks it for the reader by questioning whether born children have an inherent right to life. In the concluding sentence, they identify where they believe the emphasis should be placed in determining life or death for the newborn:

> However, if a disease has not been detected during the pregnancy, if something went wrong during the delivery, or if economical, social

> or psychological circumstances change such that taking care of the offspring becomes an unbearable burden on someone, then people should be given the chance of not being forced to do something they cannot afford.[115]

So, if "taking care of offspring" represents "an unbearable burden on someone" then infanticide—the intentional killing of that parent's child—should be a morally (and one assumes, legally) available option. Why wouldn't the same logic apply to young children, adolescents, teens, or elderly parents? If one cannot afford to keep such persons (they are, after all, the unintended products of maturation) housed and fed, why not just kill them (or perhaps more acceptably, cause the cessation of cellular biological activity)?

Making It Easy

"Abortion" is a general term that its advocates use to obscure the nature and target of that procedure. Conversely, "intentional child-killing" provides shocking clarity. When an abortion is performed, it intentionally kills a child. Anyone who hears that phrase knows precisely what is happening and to whom. In order to further obscure the true nature of elective abortion, advocates and industry mouthpieces have made a language pivot of their own. In the next chapter, you may be amazed to find that after years of hiding behind the positive word "choice," abortion advocates are publicly embracing "abortion," associating it with "normalcy," "love," and arguing that child killing is a net positive. Read on.

CHAPTER 6

Why Abortion Isn't 'Health Care' and Other Language Issues

For many years, abortion advocates tried to avoid the word "abortion." It seemed risky to use a word that focused attention on the targets, methods, or aftermath of abortion. Instead, the abortion lobby landed on the word "choice," a sound rhetorical strategy. Then, something changed among abortion advocates, they became aware that their subtle language had compromising undertones. Let's look at the evolution of "choice," the shift to "pro-abortion," the claim that "abortion is health care," and then the return to the tactic of obscuring with "reproductive freedom" and "agency." You will see how the new abortion industry language lacks the simple clarity of the term "intentional child-killing."

'Choice' Issues

In general, people like to have choices, and recoil from having their choices restricted. "Choosy mothers choose Jif" declared a common peanut butter brand campaign. For decades, parents pushed their politicians for school "choice." For many years, bumper stickers encouraged readers to "Go to the Church of Your Choice." Who could object to being "pro-choice"? Wouldn't objecting make you "anti-choice"? Abortionists focused on the freedom provided by "choices" without explicitly identifying what behaviors followed the choice-making.

Once the target of choices is made explicit, it is easy to see how the term "choice" fails to help people make moral decisions. Some actions should never be chosen: committing adultery, for example. Other actions are prohibited by law. While people still have the "choice" to engage in such behaviors, they do so at the risk of being shunned or even imprisoned. Who would ever use "choice" language to whitewash behaviors such as slavery, rape, carjacking, or burning down a neighbor's house?

Similarly, no one should be allowed to choose to intentionally kill a child, any more than someone should have a choice to intentionally have sex with a child through child sex trafficking. As already noted, organizations opposed to child sex trafficking call it exactly what it is: child sex with adults for money. No one would publicly promote child sex trafficking. You would never say, "Well, I would never personally pay to have sex with a child, but I'm not going to shove my morality down someone else's throat."

But abortion had always been a "silent subject," a topic that polite people simply didn't discuss. Substituting the positive term "choice" for the morally and emotionally loaded word "abortion" papered over the tension.

While the euphemism "choice" still pops up in speeches by political candidates, who have no alternative but to appeal to multi-generational voters, some of those actively involved in the abortion industry no longer feel the need to hide it. Abortion, in certain circles, is right out in the open.

Pro-Choice or Pro-Abortion?

If I had called my opponents "pro-abortion" when I first became involved in pro-life messaging (or "pro-abort" for short), they would have collectively lost their minds. Even recently, in a social media exchange on abortion, I had a college professor respond to me with the message: "It's pro-choice. No one is pro-abortion."

Planned Parenthood disagrees.

Planned Parenthood's action webpage instructs the organization's supporters in "appropriate" attitudes and language regarding abortion. It identifies some of the terms people use when discussing abortion and highlights the following as an example of "abortion stigma":

- "No one is pro-abortion."
- "I'm pro-choice, not pro-abortion."

Planned Parenthood's response? "Typically it's people who are supportive of abortion rights who use these phrases, but they both imply that abortion is a bad thing. It's 100% fine to support abortion—be proud to be pro-abortion."[116]

Still, many abortion advocates, particularly politicians, remain uncomfortable with the word "abortion" unless a modifier or an explanation accompanies it. Dr. Colleen McNicholas, Chief Medical Officer of Planned Parenthood of St. Louis, in a Senate Committee hearing on July 12, 2022, called on the Biden administration to declare a national health emergency in response to the *Dobbs* decision. In defiance of all rational analysis, she argued that being against abortion is "anti-life." She concluded, "Abortion is normal, it is an act of love, and it is fundamentally health care."[117]

Such testimony is possible only if one believes preborn children to be tumors or parasites, or that pregnancy is a disease rather than what it really is. The truth is that children are the natural outcome of some acts of sexual intercourse and that pregnancy is a normal biological and relational condition. Abortion advocates manipulate language in an attempt to frame abortion as "normal, loving, health care," when in fact it is the intentional, violent killing of an innocent human child.

Is Abortion Normal?

Is abortion "normal," as Dr. McNicholas suggests? Abortion may be *common*; we have killed more than sixty-five million children since 1973 in the U.S. alone, but it is not *normal.* Slavery used to be common in the U.S. (and remains so in many countries), but it is not normal.

The abnormality of abortion can be readily understood simply by reading what happens during an abortion. Martin Haskell, a notorious late-term abortionist, describes one kind of abortion (currently outlawed) that many abortion advocates would like to see reinstated: the D&X abortion.

> [T]he surgeon takes a pair of blunt curved Metzenbaum scissors in the right hand. He carefully advances the tip, curved down, along the spine and under his middle finger until he feels it contact the base of the skull under the tip of his middle finger.... [T]he surgeon then forces the scissors into the base of the skull or into the foramen magnum. Having safely entered the skull, he spreads the scissors to enlarge the opening. The surgeon removes the scissors and introduces a suction catheter into this hole and evacuates the skull contents.

Abortion is technologically invasive and physically violent. It often dismembers or poisons the bodies of preborn children who, up until that point, were safely, naturally/normally developing in the wombs of their mothers.

Children developing in their mother's wombs is *natural*; abortion is *unnatural.* And it's certainly not *normal.*

Is Abortion Loving?

Abortion is not a loving action; it has spawned an industry that preys upon desperate women, telling them that the death of their children is the price they must pay to access "the good life." No moral person who has ever seen an abortion could call it a loving action.

Abortionist Warren Hern's staff (story above) certainly didn't experience it that way. But it certainly is an action. Above and beyond any political, moral, and even spiritual *issue*, abortion is primarily an *action.* It's an action that intentionally produces casualties, a claim easy to demonstrate. All you have to do is watch videos of abortion and its aftermath.

"Loving others" means to have their best interests at heart. There is no social, economic, or relational difficulty for which the death of an innocent third person is ever the moral or loving response.

Is Abortion 'Fundamentally Health Care'?

The emphasized portion of McNicholas' remarks—the modifier "fundamentally" was added in the oral testimony—gives you the clear language path that those arguing for intentional child killing intend to take. A few examples will suffice. CNN, on July 6, 2023, described the effect of the pro-life protection laws in Texas:

> A strict abortion law that took effect in Texas in 2021 may have led to nearly 10,000 more births than expected in the last nine months of 2022, according to research published in the journal JAMA... "There were still a lot of people who were going further afield for abortion care or who were self-managing their abortion," said Bell [Suzanne Bell, the co-author of the study], who studies patterns of contraceptive use and abortion. "But our results suggest that not everyone was able to overcome those barriers, and many were forced [to carry] an unwanted or unsafe pregnancy to term."[118]

Note the term "abortion care" and how it contrasts with the clearly intended negative idea of bringing "an unwanted or unsafe pregnancy to term." I have questions. Were the 10,000 women pregnant? Yes, indeed they were. What is the natural outcome when there are 10,000 pregnant women, seeing as pregnancy is a temporary condition? Well, after approximately 40-weeks gestation, that temporary condition ends with the birth of about 10,000 babies. In other words, not having abortions led to 10,000 pregnant women giving birth to their own children. That's not exactly a shocker.

Why should that be "unexpected"? It's unexpected only if you think of child killing as the preferred alternative to all these living children. The authors expect that if individuals want to intentionally kill their children, no barrier should be placed in their way that might lead to live childbirth.

> Abortion advocates rely on an Orwellian use of language. No action can be called "health care" which has, as its preferred outcome, the intentional killing of innocent human children.

The American Journal of Obstetrics and Gynecology references "live birth" as a "risk" associated with over eleven percent of second-trimester abortions.[119] In other words, elective abortion was treated as nothing more than any other kind of medical procedure. The baby (which is what a "live birth" produces) is identified as the unintended and undesirable outcome of that medical procedure. The essay further explains how the abortionist can significantly reduce the risk and lessen the chances that a living child will emerge from the womb, an organ specifically designed to house and nurture that child: "feticidal injection may protect against this outcome" (with "this outcome" functioning as the dehumanizing term used instead of "the birth of a healthy human baby"). [120]

Consider the use of the term "feticide" by the authors. Homicide literally means "man killing." "Senicide" refers to the crime of killing the elderly (often, once they are considered burdens). People who murder their newborns are charged with "infanticide." In the case of this article from a well-regarded medical journal, "feticide" is used to describe a drug designed to intentionally kill children in the womb. Killing toddlers is murder; killing preborn children is "medicine" – that is what the abortion industry is trying to train you to believe.

Appearing on the American College of Obstetricians and Gynecologists website is an FAQ page titled "Abortion Care." Were you to click and read through the PDF, you would never encounter the words embryo, fetus, baby, or child. It describes abortion as a medical procedure designed to "empty the uterus" or "remove the pregnancy," but the page refuses to acknowledge what (much less "who") is currently occupying that space and is the target for removal.[121]

When you read language about "removing the pregnancy" or evacuating "pregnancy tissue" you are being exposed to a propaganda campaign designed to manipulate language to dehumanize human children growing in their mothers' wombs. The National Institute of Child Health and Human Development defines "pregnancy" as "a period of up to 41 weeks in which a fetus develops inside a woman's womb" and "Pregnancy is the term used to describe the period in which a fetus develops inside a woman's womb or uterus."[122] In other words, pregnancy is a time period or a condition; it is not an object that can be removed. Removing "pregnancy tissue" would be equivalent to going to a psychiatrist to have "anxiety tissue" removed. There isn't any. Anxiety, like pregnancy, is a *condition*, not a physical being.

Elective abortion is not health care. You might as well call child trafficking "asset management." In both uses, the terms "health care" or "asset management," the victim remains unnamed and unacknowledged. The *condition* of pregnancy may be attended by health-oriented complications, such as preeclampsia, gestational diabetes, or placenta previa. But pregnancy itself is not a disease, and preborn children are not tumors or parasites. Intentionally killing living, growing, innocent human beings is not health care.

Reproductive Freedom and Reproductive Justice

On February 21, 2023, California Governor Gavin Newsom announced the formation of the Reproductive Freedom Alliance, composed of twenty state governors working together to advance abortion advocacy. Currently, twenty-three governors are members.

> The alliance is now headed by Christina Chang, who worked for the nation's largest abortion business, Planned Parenthood, as both the Vice-President of Public Affairs and the Chief External Affairs Officer in New York City. Newsom's office explained the mission:
>
> The Alliance will work together to strengthen reproductive freedom in the face of an unprecedented assault on abortion access and other forms of reproductive health care by states hostile to abortion rights and judges who are advancing their ideological agenda. All Governors who support reproductive freedom are welcome to join the Alliance.[123]

On its official website, the Reproductive Freedom Alliance makes sure that readers know that the group is "nonpartisan" and that "The Reproductive Freedom Alliance is the only entity supporting and organizing Governors in the fight for fundamental reproductive freedom."[124] All twenty-three governors in the RFA are members of the Democratic Party, so it is hard to see how this alliance could be deemed "nonpartisan." No one holding to any significant position that would protect the lives of children in the womb would be admitted. Abortion without exception or gestational limitations is the official position of the Democratic Party.

"Reproductive Freedom" is also an odd term to use for an organization that wants either to encourage people not to reproduce, or to furnish the means by which parents can intentionally kill the offspring they already have reproduced. The purpose of abortion on demand is not to make people "free to reproduce." If there were truth in organizational names, this would be called the Freedom to Kill Preborn Children Alliance. Apparently, states opposing the intentional killing of innocent human beings in the womb (those very beings who provide evidence that a couple *has* "reproduced") and encouraging couples to become parents, are deemed by the RFA to be "hostile to essential reproductive health care." (Note again the use of "fundamental" and "essential" as modifiers of abortion masquerading as "health care.") Similarly, appeals to "reproductive justice" have nothing at all to do with being free to reproduce. In fact, human beings have successfully (one might say "freely") reproduced for millennia without any support or aid from government "reproductive freedom" alliances. Reproductive justice groups, such as In Our Own Voice: National Black Women's Reproductive Justice Agenda, also care little about justice as it pertains to defenseless children in the womb. In Our Own Voice declares that they are in favor of women having "the right to have children," but also "the right to not have children."[125]

Having children is a biological reality for many women, but it is not a "right." No one has a right to "have" (as in "possess," or even to "produce") a child. If, sadly, some women cannot conceive and bear children, they have no guaranteed right to possess a child conceived and born by someone else. Current debates over in-vitro fertilization and surrogacy point out the moral problems associated with some current medical technologies. In-vitro fertilization (IVF), for example, intentionally creates children only to dispose of "unwanted extras."

And what of the "right to not have children"? Pregnant women already have children. The answer for not wanting to create children is to avoid the action that gives rise to their creation. But the first order of justice should be the protection of innocent powerless human beings from other, more powerful human beings intent on exterminating them. There is no justice in killing innocent children who arise from adults engaging in reproductive freedom.

A Word on 'Access' and 'Agency'

In the same Senate hearing cited above, Senator Diane Feinstein brought up the concept of "abortion access," as it might pertain to states which choose to pass life-affirming legislation. "Access" in this case is another example of using a "virtue word," a term that denotes something principled and ethically acceptable. Everyone wants to have "access" in general, and no one wants to be "denied access." The underlying idea is that something valuable is, or should be, available to you, and it would be unjust for you to be kept from taking advantage of that good.

No one (or, thankfully, very few individuals) talk about "prostitution access" or "suicide access." Prostitution and suicide are generally identified as sexually, culturally, and morally impermissible throughout most of the U.S.[126] Once "abortion" is conflated with the terms "medical procedure" or "health care," however, the word "access" suddenly does all the heavy lifting.

Again, if the proponents of abortion argued for access to physicians who would intentionally kill their children, or access to "feticide" or drugs designed to annihilate children in the womb, far fewer people would have positive feelings toward the "access" such a policy position would provide.

Khiara Bridges, a UC Berkeley law professor, under questioning by Senator John Cornyn at the same Senate hearing, refused to ascribe any value to preborn children. In fact, she would not acknowledge their existence (stunning in light of her denunciations of Senator Josh Hawley later in the hearing. She claimed the senator was engaging in "violence" against trans people because he refused to assent to the idea that "men can be pregnant"—a refusal that in her mind meant that he denied the very existence of trans people). When Cornyn asked her if children born alive have value, Bridges paused for three full seconds, as if she had to carefully consider her answer, and then admitted they do. When Cornyn then asked if children "not yet born" have value, Bridges' response was, in a word, non-responsive. Instead, she repeated for the second time in as many minutes, "I believe that a person with a capacity for pregnancy has value, they have intelligence, they have agency..." When Cornyn reminded her that he was "talking about the baby," Bridges reasserted that she was "talking about the person with the capacity for pregnancy." When Cornyn accused her of not answering the question, she retorted that she was "answering a more interesting question."[127]

Bridges' repeated reference to "agency" echoes the appeal to "access." "Agency" simply means the ability to do something. There is nothing magical about it. Everyone has it; Bridges' "belief" is not required for you to have it.

Additionally, laws do not have the power to prohibit agency. The fact that people break the law daily demonstrates that fact. Enforcement of those laws—placing someone in jail, for instance—is specifically designed to inhibit or eliminate the willingness of people to engage in certain kinds of agency.

Three questions need answers: How is agency to be used? Are there certain acts which, even though a person has the capacity to do them, ought not to be done? And should people be prohibited by law from doing such acts?

A Final Thought on Words

"Freedom," "justice," "health care," "access," and "agency' are not terms designed to stand on their own. These words and phrases reference something outside themselves and you should be curious about what that might be. These terms need to be interrogated. When you hear them, you should reflexively ask, "freedom to do what?" "What activity are people asserting is 'just'?" "What behaviors does this person say constitute 'health care"? "To what activities should people receive free access?" "Are *all* actions, including the action to intentionally kill one's own children, appropriate ends of human agency?"

If you want to have a meaningful discussion regarding abortion, you must clearly understand and articulate *what* or *who* is the target of the action called "abortion." If no human beings are at risk, if abortion is akin to removing a diseased kidney, then I can't understand why anyone would need alliances or freedom to enable them to have access and agency to remove them. Everyone intuitively knows that removing diseased organs is the kind of action that is both permissible and encouraged. If someone wanted to keep a segment of the population infected by diseased kidneys, I suppose then they might need to seek justice, because other people were trying to harm them.

But if the target of an abortion is an innocent human being—and abortion is specifically designed to intentionally kill children—then no appeal to freedom or justice is warranted. Alliances formed to promote it are unjust, immoral, and evil. And the law should prohibit those who seek to kill their preborn neighbors from gaining access to the means of exterminating them or encouraging others to engage their agency to do so.

Public discussion regarding abortion will bear much better fruit if you and I refer to it simply by what it does.

Elective abortion is intentional child killing.

PIVOT 2

FROM APATHETIC IGNORANCE TO INTENTIONAL EDUCATION

CHAPTER 7

Learning from Our Opponents About Overcoming Ignorance

Standing in front of three dozen pastors, it seemed almost ludicrous to say it out loud. But I had to: "We now live in a time where we must teach our people not to intentionally kill their own children." It's a weird thing to say to pastors, right?

Isn't it obvious that people shouldn't intentionally kill their own children? It should go without saying. Unfortunately, many in church leadership have gone for decades without saying it.

The silence has persisted for so long that young people, raised in the church, graduate from high school without ever hearing a well-reasoned, comprehensive argument for why intentionally killing children is wrong. Then they go on, perhaps, to a Christian college where, after four years (culminating in a diploma, maybe even graduating with a degree in pastoral ministry) they never encounter a developed pro-life apologetic. Some of those students enter seminary, and after three or more years of grueling work, having learned complex theology and at least a rudimentary reading level of Greek and Hebrew, they receive their Master of Divinity degree.

And yet, during that entire academic journey, never once were they required to read any of the many books exploring the scientific, philosophical, or theological underpinnings of the pro-life position and how best to respond to the advocates of intentional child-killing.

These new pastors enter into the life of the church as leaders and teachers, but nothing in their experience has prepared them to defend the proposition that abortion is a grave moral evil. I daresay that most of them intuitively believe that people engaging in the intentional killing of children are doing something unspeakably immoral and wrong. Unfortunately, too many are ill-equipped to explain *why*. No one taught them. It was assumed they just knew it.

But assumptions won't protect the flock against carefully-crafted propaganda or against pro-abortion philosophical positions that are strange, new, and which feed people's self-interest. It's an alluring proposition to be told that you should be able to do whatever you want with your own body.

Unfortunately, today's churches are filled with Christians who are easy targets for abortion advocates. I don't necessarily mean that all these people could be persuaded to take the lives of their own children (though the abortion statistics on church-going Christians are grim). What I do mean is that the ignorance of believers puts them in intellectual and moral peril.

You need to understand this cycle of educational silence—and the cycle continues to repeat—so that you can grasp how the church finds itself in this mess. In *Contenders*, I explore eight reasons why pastors don't (or don't often or effectively) preach on abortion. One reason is ignorance of the topic; but until recently, I hadn't thought much about why that is the case. Many pastors and teachers operate out of ignorance because no one, and I mean not one person during all their formative and formal educational years, ever instructed them. That is a shame. I have dedicated a fair amount of my professional life to trying to remedy that informational deficit by directly training pastors. This chapter explores three topics:

- Why avoiding discussions of important topics, especially out of fear, hurts the ignorant
- The educational disadvantages faced by the pro-life movement
- How the other side uses education and what pro-life advocates can learn from it

Avoidance Invites Dissent

Ignorance, by intention or neglect, never strengthens anyone. It simply makes the introduction of heretical or immoral ideas novel and, therefore, more interesting and even compelling.

Deconstruction, where Christians re-examine and question sometimes long-held beliefs, is a prime example of a spiritual problem born of ignorance coupled with a lack of solid answers. Some in the church are waking up and many are marshalling efforts to respond. But churches unwilling to do the hard work of introducing young people to tough ideas through a purposeful course of study, open discussion, and debate, invited deconstructionists to win their victories.

As a result, few young Christians are biblically literate, know how to handle difficult passages of Scripture, feel comfortable with some aspects of the mystery of God (for example, that some knowledge is hidden from humans), faith, and uncertainty, or understand much about science (how it is done, how it is used, and its limitations). A TikTok generation of winsome, individual subject-matter experts are free to sow internal discord and doubt in the minds of the unprepared (and now, perhaps, former) believers. Instead of grounding Christians, many pastors find themselves on the defensive, trying to justify doctrines previously thought to be unassailable. Instead of defending solid ground, some are trying to backfill craters in their faith.

Similarly, if churches are unwilling or unable to teach a coherent sexual ethic that demonstrates understanding of the arguments marshalled against it, and have prepared thoughtful, persuasive responses, then they should not feel surprised that their young people not only fall into sexual sin but embrace it as a new identity. If believers are not grounded in the scientific, moral, and biblical case for life in a way that directly confronts the alternative positions that abortion advocates make, they will be easy prey.

Wait a Minute! What About the Pro-Life Movement?

The pro-life movement is older than *Roe v. Wade*. For many decades, a host of organizations have been teaching the truth about the sanctity of human life. These tireless advocates have sponsored educational campaigns, published books, written articles in scholarly journals and for popular periodicals, created blogs, podcasts, posted videos, spoken from stages, engaged in debates, and worked through one-on-one conversations with students on campus and with people in the streets. With all that interaction, wouldn't you think that the people would certainly know by now what the pro-life view is? Is it possible that they are just tired of hearing about it?

Not remotely.

For starters, the number of individuals in the life-affirming education space is small, compared to the chokehold the public educational system has on each successive generation. Mainstream media, and not just the news but also entertainment and social platforms, has a virtual lock on internal culture creation. And the law, which for decades across this nation has functioned as a tutor of death, still today erases offspring and champions abortion in far too many states. By funding and advocating that nothing valuable exists in the womb of a pregnant woman—they won't even admit the child's existence—states lead their people to believe that women who rid themselves of "pregnancy tissue" are exercising their right to "comprehensive health care." One entire major political party incessantly beats the pro-abortion drum and marches in lockstep, while the other party *may* talk a bit about abortion whenever election time rolls around. Finally, many private organizations evangelize with the gospel of abortion. They argue that sacrificing your children can be the key to attaining the good life you desire and deserve.

The educational output of the entire pro-life movement is a whisper seeking a hearing amid the cacophony of popular culture. As my pro-life colleague, Gregg Cunningham, once observed, the bottom line is that your opponents are more committed to killing children than the rest of the nation is to saving them.

That didn't happen overnight. Neither will its reversal. With apologies to G.K. Chesterton, pro-life education has not been tried and found wanting; it has been found difficult (and uncomfortable) and left (largely) untried.[128]

When I teach a three-hour pro-life apologetics course at churches throughout the U.S., I frequently ask my audiences, "How many of you have ever heard a comprehensive case for life like the one you listened to this evening?" Most of the time, no one raises a hand. When I spoke last year in Kansas, only three people raised their hands: one was Catholic, while the other two were Orthodox. Not a single evangelical Protestant raised a hand. Rather than feel discouraged, let's accept this sad state of affairs as a challenge.

To Tell the Truth

Much of the problem regarding inoculating Christians against the persuasive propaganda of pro-abortion forces is a crippling shyness that teachers in many churches have about making strong truth claims. Harry Blamires noted this way back in 1965. Speaking like a prophet who saw an era where the greatest sin would be certainty, he wrote:

> Yet in every other religious journal one picks up to-day one reads the amazing sentence: 'We must not talk as though we've got all the answers.' Why, in God's name not? What is our Christian duty if not to make plain that in the Christian Faith the gravest doubts and worries of men are richly answered?...The supposed duty of the Christian to take shelter behind a veil of incomprehensibility is an invention of the Devil.[129]

Too many "seeker-friendly" churches forget that seeking is not an end in itself; the purpose of seeking is to find. Some people say, "the journey's the thing," but that's not remotely true. The purpose of a journey is to reach a desired destination. If you don't know and don't mind not knowing where you are going or where you are, you are the functional definition of being lost.

People ask questions because they want answers. As a rhetorician, I understand that locating absolute certainty in answers for many questions is difficult, if not impossible. But most people are looking for answers that are reasonable, probable, defensible, better justified than alternatives, and based in the best available evidence. Most Christians would claim that the arguments supporting the resurrection of Jesus Christ meet these standards. The scientific and moral claims regarding the nature and value of children in the womb do so as well.

There is always room for doubt and debate on every significant question. But some fundamental questions have clear answers. We should be unafraid and unashamed to give them.

Human life begins at conception; everything after is just human development. Abortion is an act of violence that intentionally kills a preborn child. Intentionally killing innocent human beings is wrong. These are medical and moral facts. (If you don't believe that moral facts exist, read C.S. Lewis' book *The Abolition of Man* and he will explain them to you.)

The first challenge Christians must face in educating others about the sanctity of human life and the evil of abortion is to honestly believe they have something true to say. The second challenge is developing the courage to say it. Courageous education, that is, teaching that doesn't shrink from the arguments of those who stridently object, can make a difference. And you will find this to be true even when the subject matter is highly polarizing, peer-group popular, and deeply emotional. Consider one case in point.

A Geography Lesson

After the horrific slaughter, rape and kidnapping of Israeli citizens on October 7, 2023, at the hands of Hamas militants who overran the Nova music festival, college campuses all over the United States erupted in protest. Not against Hamas, the terrorist organization that was/is the elected government of the Gaza region, but in support of it. "From the river to the sea, Palestine must be free" chanted thousands of university students, some waving Palestinian flags and wearing Palestinian keffiyehs.

Ron Hassner, professor of political science at UC Berkeley, wanted to know on what basis these students engaged in such robust rhetoric. He hired a firm to survey 250 students from across the U.S.. He discovered that more than half the students chanting this slogan could not identify the river (the Jordan River) or the sea (the Mediterranean Sea). They were ignorant about the land mass in question.[130]

He showed eighty students a map of the region and explained that if Palestinians were to be free from the river to the sea, it would mean that Israeli citizens would have no place to live. The result? Three quarters of these students "downgraded" their "enthusiasm for the mantra to 'probably not'." Additionally, "Sixty percent of those students reduced their support for the slogan when they learned it would entail the subjugation, expulsion or annihilation of seven million Jewish and two million Arab Israelis."[131]

The encouraging conclusion of this research project was that 67.8 percent of the students who had been in favor of the slogan, now rejected it. So, why had they been so vocal in support? Hassner doesn't offer a rationale, but it's not hard to imagine that many students had engaged in groupthink. They wanted to go do something exciting and revel in being counter-cultural. Hassner does reveal that the students were ignorant. Many had never seen a map of the area and knew little to nothing about the issue they had so passionately advocated.

The final two sentences in Hassner's essay are particularly illuminating: "Those who hope to encourage extremism depend on the political ignorance of their audiences. It is time for good teachers to join the fray and combat bias with education."[132]

Accept the challenge.

Our Opponents Play This Game

A big problem faced California back in 2022. More precisely, it had a Big 10 problem. In 2016, the California state legislature, aided by Governor Jerry Brown, passed and signed into law Assembly Bill 1887, which banned state-funded travel to any state deemed to have anti-LGBTQ laws in place. At first, the policy affected only a handful of states; but soon it grew to seventeen, eventually peaking at twenty-three—nearly half of the U.S.[133]

In 2022, UCLA Football announced it was leaving the Pac-12 to join the more prestigious Big 10 Conference.[134] There was just one slight hiccup. The Indiana Hoosiers, the Purdue Boilermakers (Indiana), the Iowa Hawkeyes, and the Ohio State Buckeyes all hailed from states on the blacklist. That meant that UCLA Football could not use state money to travel to any away games against any of those four teams. What could an enterprising coaching staff do?

Scott Markley, then the senior associate athletic director at the school (now working for the Big 10 Conference), was asked how UCLA football would manage to go to away games while complying with the law. He gave a telling response:

> Should UCLA compete or recruit in a banned state, in compliance with the law, none of the costs for travel to that state will come from state funds. In addition, if a team competes in a banned state, student-athletes and staff will receive education about the relevant California law, the law at issue in the destination state, and given the choice to opt out of the travel with no risk of consequence.[135]

Reread that last sentence and remember it. It will be important later.

Once the number of banned states threatened to eclipse the number of approved states, California saw the economic writing on the wall and began working to repeal the boycott. In 2023, California Senate President pro Tempore Toni Atkins introduced SB447. This proposed legislation didn't merely repeal the boycott of conservative states which dared to oppose California's position on gender ideology and perverse sexual ethics; it strategically replaced it. As *Los Angeles Times* columnist Nicholas Goldberg explained:

> Although she initially voted for the ban back in 2016, Atkins now believes it's time for a "pivot," as she put it, because "polarization is not working." She hopes to repeal the boycott and replace it with a California-sponsored publicity campaign in red states to encourage LGBTQ acceptance and discourage discrimination.[136]

Atkins wants education at home and a programmed campaign of persuasion away. As noted in the first chapter, exporting abortion messaging to pro-life states is nothing new for California. Gavin Newsom demonstrated it through his interstate pro-abortion billboard campaign.

People claim that they would rush into a burning building to save a child. I assume these same people teach their own children not to play with matches. Surely, then, to save children from an avoidable death, we should be willing to educate our young people against the danger of abortion.

SB447 was signed into law in 2023, establishing the "Building and Reinforcing Inclusive and Diverse, Gender-Supportive Equity Project" (BRIDGE). Goldberg explained why he favored this bill, despite fellow progressives who argued, "there's little to be gained from discussions with conservatives, evangelicals or bigots who simply can't be reasoned with."[137] He believes that people should dialogue over their differences. And when he says "people" he means that his side should use the power of the state.

The text of SB447 is instructive.[138] BRIDGE functions out of the governor's office and is tasked with, among other things, not promoting "a political purpose." But in the following paragraph:

> (2) Media campaigns may be on a national scale and, to the extent possible, may target audiences in a state or states, or a media market that includes a state or states that have enacted a law that voids or repeals, or has the effect of voiding or repealing, an existing state or local protection against discrimination on the basis of sexual orientation, gender identity, or gender expression, or have enacted a law that authorizes or requires discrimination against same-sex couples or their families or on the basis of sexual orientation, gender identity, or gender expression, including any law that creates an exemption to antidiscrimination laws in order to permit discrimination against same-sex couples or their families or on the basis of sexual orientation, gender identity, or gender expression.[139]

The BRIDGE Advisory Council is *required* to have LGBTQ+ advocates as members. So, in California, the perceived objective moral truth undergirding LGBTQ+ ideology is so universal that promoting it openly in states that have rejected it doesn't count as "political."

At the time of this writing, no reports have surfaced about the amount of funding BRIDGE has received from the Governor's Office. Neither have I been able to discover any media campaigns issued by BRIDGE, or even who makes up the committee. The inability to discover the funding, work, or who has been appointed to a ten-member advisory committee embedded in the California governor's office should be problematic for any California taxpayer; but in the Golden State, fiscal irregularities and shady deals are commonplace. Alternately, it could be that the legislation was just for show, and, like California's high-speed train, is going nowhere.

My point is not to identify ghost committees or to ferret out funding. I want to demonstrate that powerful states don't shy away from using the government to advance what they perceive to be, however wrongheaded, the policy of *their* state into *other* states that disagree. Rather than bury you in analysis, I want to show you an educational model, one these states can hardly object to if they are currently doing it themselves.

Why Education Comes First

The citizens of deeply conservative states may wonder aloud, "But how are we going to get our schools to agree to do this?" I'll address how to legislatively implement these proposals and others later. For now, just understand that the political lens through which many pro-life people view the fact of intentional child-killing often leads them to believe that the only meaningful answers come from the government. But there is a reason why this chapter on education comes before the chapter on legislation.

GOTV vs. GITV

You may have heard the term GOTV; it stands for Get Out The Vote. You know, canvass your neighborhood, drive like-minded voters to the polls, work phone banks, remind people to mail in their absentee ballots, get everyone likely to vote with you to actually do so. GOTV relies on corralling people who are already persuaded, or at least heavily inclined, to agree with you. Those who win locate their own voters most effectively and then get them to the polls. GOTV efforts tend to be frantic, talk in sound bites, and depend on emotional appeals—a whipping behavior. GOTV doesn't allow for deep explanations of public policy or even winning over detractors. The goal is not to educate but to motivate to act.

While political parties rely on GOTV, pro-life advocates have a more complex and important mission: GITV, or Get In The Voter. You can't wait to do this until right before election day. In fact, because untimely pregnancy can always be "right around the corner," it's best not to delay at all. Your children and all the people in your community need to know the truth. They need to grounded in the ethics of life. That way, when they find out that they or a friend are experiencing an untimely pregnancy, they'll know what to say and how to act.

And there's a bonus. If you do a solid job educating your children, grounding them in a defensible pro-life apologetic, you will inoculate them against abortion advocacy. No one will have to pull out cattle prods to drive them to vote when they become adults. People trained to have consistent scientific, moral, and biblical worldviews know what to do.

What Pro-Life States Can Learn from California

Do you remember that second sentence from UCLA's former assistant athletic director, Scott Markley? He unwittingly laid out precisely the plan that pro-life states must implement. Here it is: 1) teach students about the relevant law in their state; 2) teach students about the law in the destination state. Markley declared that California intends to use inoculation theory on their student athletes. The good news is that inoculation theory will work exceptionally well in pro-life states.

The other encouraging note is that the inoculation intended by Markley will not be as effective as he thought it would be when students from pro-life states visit California. In fact, in order to maintain their grip on the pro-abortion imaginations of their young people, they will need to keep them as far as possible from the truth about pro-life laws and their scientific and philosophical underpinnings. For people with pro-abortion worldviews, contact with their opponent carries a titanic risk of "infection."

Inoculation and How It Works

Most people know how medical inoculation works. A dead or weakened form of a virus is introduced into the body, triggering the creation of antibodies to fight off the initial infection. Then, when a real viral attack comes, the body is prepared. Just as you can inoculate against disease, so you can inoculate against ideas. The steps are very similar.

If you want to convince people to believe some truth claim that they have been enculturated to see as false, you don't directly leap in with counter-claims and evidence. That strategy will likely only stiffen your opponent's resistance. Instead, frame the argument/discussion this way:

1. Respectfully explain your opponent's position(s).
2. Using reasoning, analysis, and evidence, demonstrate that your opponent's position(s) is (are) flawed.
3. Explain your position by making claims and providing superior evidence.
4. Identify the impact of the argument. If X is their position—if X is unjustifiable and indefensible and if your position is superior—then ask how people should believe, think and/or act about that subject.

In the example about the pro-Palestinian student protesters, the researchers identified the opponent's position: "From the river to the sea, Palestine must be free." The protesters agreed that they supported this slogan. The researchers then demonstrated that many of the protesters didn't know what the slogan meant. Pulling out a map, the researchers showed the protesters the actual geographical layout of Israel and explained that if the slogan were enacted, it would annihilate or displace millions of Israeli Jews and Arabs. Finally, they revisited the slogan with the protesters, and the vast majority of students who, minutes earlier, had been committed enough to chant it in the streets, now rejected it. I'm guessing that they will not rejoin such protests in the future.

Now consider a popular cultural position in the abortion "controversy": what's in a woman's body at the moment of conception isn't a human being. I don't want to create a straw man of that position. I don't want to misrepresent my opponent's position for the purpose of making it easier to attack. I also want to make it clear that most professional abortion advocates know and will admit, if pressed, that there *is* a human being in the womb of a pregnant mother. By contrast, the position most abortion supporters take is that while the child is technically *human*, it's not actually a *person*. But the idea that the child is not a human being is popularly held.

To ensure accuracy, I'll use evidence to demonstrate that I accurately picture what pro-abortion advocates claim. I can look to Planned Parenthood's own website which, in describing aspiration abortion, never once mentions the target of the abortion.[140] Instead, it refers to the living, distinct child in the womb with the dehumanizing language of "the pregnancy." I might show videos of college students yelling "It's a fetus!" when a pro-life advocate accurately describes the being in the mother's womb as a "child" or a "baby." I'll use Katha Pollit's abortion advocacy book *Pro*, to show how she argues that for weeks after conception, the child in the womb is just too small to count as a human being worth protecting.[141] Senator Dick Durbin echoed that idea in a Senate hearing in 2023 when he said, "In my mind, this gets to the heart of the issue and the debate. When does life begin? The debate has been going on for a long period of time, maybe from the beginning of civilization. I'm not sure I have the right answer. I'm not sure Dr. Skop has the right answer."[142] You won't have to work too hard to convince people that abortion advocates and supporters believe preborn children are not human, because many individuals take that position for granted.

Regarding life and death issues, especially, we shouldn't too quickly accept unsupported claims without first questioning them. The human nature of the child in the womb is not hard to demonstrate. Embryologists know that human life begins at conception.[143] Geneticists know that human life begins at conception.[144] Pro-abortion doctors in the early 1970s freely admitted that human life begins at conception, but then put forth what they called "a schizophrenic sort of subterfuge" in order to hide that truth from the public.[145] Planned Parenthood used to distribute a booklet that claimed human life begins at conception.[146] It is abundantly clear that the evidence does not support the claim that what is in a woman's body from the moment of conception is not a human being.

You can then show how we know that from the earliest moment of conception until birth and beyond, a human life resides in the womb and goes through development stages that continue throughout life. Calling a human being a zygote, embryo, or fetus is no different than calling a human being a baby, a toddler, a boy or girl, a tween, a teenager, a middle-aged adult, or a senior citizen. Each stage of life represents the same human being.

Once you know the falsehood of the pro-abortion claim that human life does not begin at conception, you cite the evidence that proves the opposite, namely, that human life *does* begin at conception. And then you draw the appropriate conclusion. If it is wrong to intentionally kill innocent human beings, and if abortion intentionally kills an innocent human being, then abortion is wrong. People shouldn't engage in wrong actions. And if the wrong action results in the deaths of innocent human beings, then they shouldn't do it themselves and should work to help others see the truth and, if necessary, prevent them from doing wrong.

From Theory to Practice

From researchers to educators, you've seen that there is much to admire in a solid educational approach. But knowing that education is needed isn't the same as actively pursuing it. So, let's see what is required to deliver the kind of knowledge that stops abortion advocacy in its tracks and builds a life-affirming worldview.

CHAPTER 8

Education Action Steps

No one *intends* to have an unintended pregnancy. Such pregnancies are untimely, and as a result abortion is often an "impulse buy." The choice to intentionally kill a child in the womb will be made only according to the information people have when the crisis strikes.

Information precedes policy (or, at least, it should). We can't expect changes in our law or culture from an ignorant citizenry. We can't expect good decisions regarding unintended pregnancy if policy originates in an informational vacuum.

In this chapter, you'll see that ignorance regarding the nature of preborn children in the womb is significant. Fortunately, ignorance can be cured with information. And a solid educational campaign doesn't have to wait for government school adoption to be successful. You can begin now. The best part? Well-structured education can actually inoculate people against abortion advocacy.

Widespread Ignorance

The ignorance in our culture regarding fetal development is astounding. I surveyed more than 1,000 students coast to coast, beginning in 2010 and continuing for many years. The overwhelming majority of students did not know that human life begins at conception. Most thought human life began with the presence of brain waves or a heartbeat. Some students listed "at birth" as the beginning of life.

Watch campus videos from Mark Harrington's organization, Created Equal, or videos where Charlie Kirk dialogued with students on campus. Over and over, you will see young adults denying the presence of a human being in the womb of the mother, or if they do acknowledge the presence of a human being there, they say that the "being," "creature," or "parasite" doesn't qualify as a human person.

Clearly, students in our nation's schools aren't learning the truth about the nature of preborn children or the threat posed by abortion. Our government, including the public school system, has contributed in a major way to crafting the child-killing worldview that many students unreflectively adopt. C.S. Lewis put it like this: "It's not a theory they [immoral teachers] put into a student's mind, but an assumption, which, ten years hence, its origin forgotten and its presence unconscious, will condition him to take one side in a controversy which he has never recognized as a controversy at all."[147] To trust the conditioners responsible for the worldview you want abolished to be the ones to fix the problem would be lunacy. Our work must start at home and in the church.

People won't learn about the truth through popular mass-media outlets, from our medical community (the American College of Obstetricians and Gynecologists is on record supporting abortion on demand throughout pregnancy), or from many state governments. Waiting on public institutions to tackle the challenge only continues to imperil children in the womb.

You Don't Have to Wait

The good news is that you don't have to wait . . . but you do have to decide. You must make a commitment to the education of your own children. If you teach a small group, life group, Sunday school class, or you are a pastor in the pulpit, you can begin educating your people.

If you want to develop a solid worldview among your children, in your sphere of influence, or in your church, you will need to do so deliberately. I love what the Apostle Paul writes in Philippians 3:1: "To write the same things again is no trouble to me, and is a safeguard for you." It is no trouble to Paul because he teaches what he already knows and has taught repeatedly. It is a safeguard to his readers because repetition builds worldviews, and worldviews are the foundation for action.

Two Scenarios

Imagine two scenarios. In the first, a young woman named Emily discovers she is pregnant despite using some birth control measure. She wanted to have sexual intercourse. She doesn't want to be pregnant. She knows little to nothing about the child in her womb. Planned Parenthood has spent hundreds of millions of dollars establishing itself as the subject matter expert on sexuality and abortion. At school and in the mass media, no impediment to abortion has ever been raised. In the state where Emily lives, the government maintains a website directing her to seek out an abortion provider. Every information outlet tells her that abortion is nothing more than health care and that "the procedure" gently removes unwanted tissue from her uterus. In this way, they tell her, the pregnancy just goes away.

What is Emily likely to do? How has her life experience primed her to act?

In the second scenario, a young woman, Hailee, has been raised in a home and in a church that doesn't shy away from teaching about children in the womb and the nature of abortion. From the time she was in elementary school, she has known that human life begins at conception. She's been taught to value those little lives as fellow image-bearers of God. Additionally, Hailee's church teaches the truth about human sexuality and its place in marriage, but also that people may sin in these areas, not just by engaging in sexual activity before marriage, but through porn usage and entertaining lust. All disobedience to God's word is sin, it teaches, and all people are guilty and in need of a Savior.

There are two ways to spoil a child's innocence: by showing them or telling them things they ought not see or hear, or by directly victimizing them. Because an Enemy exists who intends to directly harm human image bearers of God, wise parents will shield their children as long as they can, but will choose to tell them about evil rather than allow them to be victimized by it.

The gospel announces the good news that people don't need to be defined by their past sins. Hailee learns by experience that confession and repentance bring forgiveness, healing, and restoration. She knows that the consequences of some sins continue even after forgiveness is received. Hailee believes that sex before marriage is a sin. She knows that sex is inherently a baby-making act and that even when people take measures against child creation, sometimes those measures fail. Children conceived outside of wedlock may be the tangible evidence of sinful behavior, her youth pastor tells her, but the children themselves are not sinful. The commitment to these truths is clear in the way the church openly supports its area PHC and in how it established an Embrace Grace program to welcome into the life of the church clients from PHCs who come to know Jesus. Hailee knows what abortion is and what it does to the body of a child in the womb. She has heard the testimony of women with abortion in their past who warn young people against intentionally killing their children. Hailee also knows the arguments of abortion advocates. She has read about them and has seen the scientific, moral, and biblical responses to those arguments.

But in her senior year of high school, in a weak moment, Hailee has sexual relations with her boyfriend. Soon afterward she discovers she is pregnant. Given the environment in which she has been raised, the knowledge that has been reinforced, and the examples she has seen—even though her pregnancy will present difficulties—what is she more likely to do?

While the outcome is never 100 percent certain, Hailee has a much better chance of making a life-affirming decision. She has been told the truth and seen how it is embodied in her church. As a result, Hailee is far less likely than Emily to make an abortion "impulse buy." The trusting relationships she has established with people who care about her and have instructed her will be right there, informing her decision.

Protecting Innocence

"What about childhood innocence? Shouldn't that be protected?" ask many families and churches. I would answer, "certainly, up to a point." You reach that point when you know that abortion advocates have directly targeted your family. To leave children defenseless would be irresponsible—and targeting starts sooner than you might think.

Planned Parenthood tries to worm its way into the minds of your kids even before kindergarten. The YouTube Channel, Amaze Jr., is connected to the nation's largest abortion business; its videos are rated 4+ on YouTube.[148] So, who's the target audience? Pre-kindergarteners.

Early videos show cartoon drawings of intimate body parts. Children are taught such things as "most girls have a vulva" and "most boys have a penis."[149] Note the modifier: "most," not "all" or just girls and boys. What are young boys to think? If only "most" boys have penises, then there must be "some" boys who don't. These videos lay the groundwork for transgender ideology—at four years old. Planned Parenthood, in addition to its abortion business, also supplies transgender hormones.[150] As kids grow older, Amaze Jr. gets replaced by Amaze, where the content gets increasingly more explicit.

By the time most students reach sixth grade, they not only transition from elementary school to junior high, they transition from being targets of influence to becoming targets for artificial birth control and abortion. Planned Parenthood works hard to establish itself as the "trusted provider" and "subject matter expert" on all things sexual. It has won numerous awards for its advertising and marketing skill. In 2019, *Fast Company* honored Planned Parenthood with its Most Innovative Company award in the education sector "for giving teens easy access to sexual health info."[151] It has become so firmly entrenched that California's Abortion Access website openly derides pregnancy help centers and clinics as "fake," while the only "trusted providers" are to be located on the "abortion finder" page, just one click away from the landing page.[152]

I understand and laud parents who want to protect their children's innocence, but many activists out there strategize to drive a wedge between parents and their children. Planned Parenthood and other sex advocacy groups don't want parents to be the authority regarding sexual matters involving minors. The battle already rages and your children are the battlefield. When attacks come, good parents can't turn a blind eye or engage in wishful thinking that the enemy's campaign won't affect their family. Wise parents see the true nature of the attack and prepare their children to turn it back.

Will keeping your kids from smartphones, monitoring their media consumption, or using web filtering technology be enough to repel bad influences? No. Young people are primed to explore and virtual private networks or proxy servers often overcome parental safeguards. Kids can do a search for "how to bypass parental controls" and discover several ways to do so. Even if parents rightfully assume that their children can't or won't access sexually subversive information on their phones or tablets, that doesn't stop them from encountering the same information at libraries or on the devices of their friends. The most effective safeguard for our children is the same approach we offer adults: correct information delivered at the appropriate time.

Structuring Defenses

Imagine the sheer number of counterfeiters in existence. Each one, to varying degrees, attempts to create currency so realistic that it can be passed off as genuine. The challenge to a cashier or bank teller is to be able to look at a $20 bill and determine whether it is real or fake.

But bank tellers don't go to counterfeit identification school. Instead, they become intimately familiar with all the details of a real bill. They know about the paper, the threads in it, its watermarks, the magnetic strip—all manner of minutiae. Each teller knows a real bill so well that any counterfeit bill, upon inspection, becomes immediately apparent. (I have never verified this common story, but it illustrates an important lesson: when you know the truth, impostors find it much harder to trick you.)

The entire pro-life argument hinges on the medical fact that human life begins at conception. Without establishing that truth, those who want to intentionally kill preborn children will create fictions to justify their actions. So, how can we instruct people in the truths undergirding the pro-life position? Simple: through a program of educational structures.

Unstructured Play

Very young girls like to play with baby dolls. In the U.S., the baby doll market is expected to grow from $10.9 billion in 2025 to $18 billion by 2035.[153] The *Financial Market Insights* report reveals the somewhat obvious reasons: "Baby dolls are a staple in children's toys, offering developmental benefits such as social skills, nurturing behaviors, and emotional intelligence through role-playing."[154]

Little boys may bristle at playing with dolls, but they, too, see parents caring for real children, as well as their playmates—little girls—mothering baby dolls. Baby dolls help little girls relate to their mothers. And for first-born girls, such dolls often represent their initial exposure to the value and fragility of babies, who must be sheltered and nurtured.

The corollary lesson for young boys is playing army or knights. Through such play, they learn that by being strong and courageous, they can protect the weak and defenseless. Nurturing and protective messaging in the home and in the church during the early years lay an important foundation.

Age-Appropriate, Life-Affirming Curriculum

While role playing as parents and protectors can create an effective cultural foundation, you still need to clearly instruct young people about the truth in order to confront pro-abortion messaging. The following provides an outline of the kinds of topics children and youth need to encounter to protect them from the persuasive propaganda of the abortion industry.

This program can be adapted for use in churches and in schools. I encourage both to do so. But individual parents should not wait for their churches or schools (private or public) to wake up to the need. It is imperative to teach this material to your children at home. Although these topic areas aren't difficult to grasp or talk about, it will require a little courage. Pray for the boldness to protect your children.

As noted in the introduction to this book, I do not intend to rewrite the apologetics material readily available in my earlier book, *Contenders*. That book also contains all the information you need to construct teaching lessons, speeches, and sermons. What follows, therefore, only touches on the topic areas you will want to address (rather than fully developing them), and the best times to talk about each.

Science Is on Our Side: Fetal Development at 6-10+

Unstructured play and role modeling build children attuned to the care and protection of the weak and defenseless. By ten years of age, or fourth grade, the time comes to move beyond mere play and dive more deeply into the science of fetal development.

As early as elementary school, we should both tell and show children in our homes and churches the truth about how human beings are created and how they develop. The discussion need not be explicit (questions about how mommy and daddy create babies can be deferred) but it should be intentional. One outstanding visual resource is popularly known as the Baby Olivia video, easily accessed online.[155]

Young people watching the video will see a sperm cell uniting with an egg cell, fusing to create little Baby Olivia. Through the ensuing weeks, viewers watch how the little girl is "knit together in her mother's womb." As she grows in size, she develops in abilities: she swallows, sucks her thumb, moves her arms and legs, and hiccups. But it's not what Olivia is able to *do* that makes her human; she *is* human and the nature of human beings is to develop these kinds of abilities.

The video ends with Olivia's birth, merely a relocation from inside her mother's womb to the outside world. Live Action, the producer of this video, offers an accompanying board book for children.[156] The animated images in the Baby Olivia video are perfect for younger children. The Education Resource Fund also has an area for young children that includes a documentary, coloring books, and games.[157]

The Visual Becomes Tactile: 10+

It's one thing to look at an image of a preborn child in the womb, it's quite another to hold one (well, it's impossible to hold one, but you can handle a replica). For years, PHCs have used fetal models as a means of connecting young people with the reality of preborn children. John Ensor's PassionLife Ministries developed the most anatomically-accurate fetal models to date. Young people who are able to handle these tiny representations are astounded at the detail. The real children imaged by the models are obviously human.

In South America, PassionLife operates as PasiónVida. Typically, the Christian school leaders, along with the local pastors, are eager for their students to learn why abortion is morally wrong and how to defend their prolife views. Recently in Colombia, PasiónVida's Anderson Ocampo spoke to seventh graders. "Many of you will one day face the question of how to respond to an unplanned pregnancy. My goal is to make the thought of having an abortion as hard as possible," I handed each student a fetal model. "Look at the tiny fingers and toes!" I invited them. "Did you know that its taste buds and all major organs have already begun to form? Isn't it amazing that your preference for chocolate was already developing when you were that small?" [158]

By showing the students how the bodies of children in the womb are delightfully intricate, he makes it difficult for them to consider intentionally ending the life of such a child. When students can clearly image the human child, when they discover affinity for them, it places another barrier in the way of abortion advocacy.

From Animation to Imaging: Fetal Development at 12+

Older children in junior or senior high can view outstanding high-quality intrauterine endoscopic videos produced by the Education Resource Fund.[159] These videos aren't animation or AI-generated, but actual, direct images of human beings growing in the wombs of their mothers. Also available for viewing are 3D models of individual embryonic and fetal organs, which the models compare to adult organs. This award-winning site has a trove of medically accurate information that establishes and reinforces the fact that human life begins at conception. Everything after that is simple continuation. The teenager or adult looking at these images knows that the human being they are today is the same human being they once were as they grew in their mother's womb.

It should be nearly impossible to persuade those exposed to these images and information that the child in the womb is not a human being. Anyone suggesting such nonsense, even to an elementary school student, would be met with a childlike, "No, it is a human being. I know." Why do they know? Because they have seen it and are familiar with it; any other claim instantly gets recognized as counterfeit.

As young people grow older, they can be introduced to scientific evidence that explains the truth they have seen in the videos. While working toward seeing accurate fetal development taught in all of our schools, anyone can go ahead and teach it *now* at home and in church.

What God Has to Say about Human Beings and Intentional Killing: 12+

Christian parents and educators can explain in greater detail what God's Word says about the nature of human beings, that they are image bearers of God.[160] Like all other living things, human beings reproduce after their own kind.[161] Human parents give birth exclusively to human children; they couldn't possibly bear any other kind of creature. Humans are "fearfully and wonderfully made," are of incalculable value, and their lives must be protected from those who would do them harm.[162]

God explicitly forbids humans from intentionally killing innocent human beings.[163] To do so is to incur "bloodguilt." That guilt extends not just to the people directly responsible for the killing, but also to those who know it is happening but do nothing to stop it.[164]

Throughout history, individuals have engaged in child sacrifice, bargaining the lives of their children to get something from an idol. In ancient Israel, these sacrifices took place in Molech worship. God calls this behavior an abomination.[165] Instead, God wants the lives of the innocent to be preserved and protected. Jesus loves children and cited them, in a lesson to His disciples, as examples of the characteristics required to enter His Kingdom.[166]

Directly Engaging Pro-Abortion Ideas: 13+

It may be hard for parents to imagine, but by the time their children hit puberty, the abortion industry already has painted targets on their backs. They see your children as customers for transgender sex hormone therapies, birth control pills and devices, and, if and when those fail, abortions. Helping young people recognize Planned Parenthood's "customer acquisition" process involves taking the mask off the arguments they advance and replacing them with the truth. These topic areas require an inoculation approach. For each topic you must:

- know what line of argument or reasoning abortion industry organizations use;
- be able to expose the flaws in their arguments, using evidence and reasoning;
- explore what is true;
- explain how knowing these arguments alters thinking, along with suggestions about what actions should be taken.

Once the student is old enough to encounter advocacy, start with an easy-to-understand argument that undergirds everything that follows. My colleague, Scott Klusendorf, calls this The Syllogism. Pro-life advocates have successfully defended it in a variety of forms for many years:

- It is wrong to intentionally kill an innocent human being
- Abortion intentionally kills an innocent human being
- Therefore, abortion is wrong

Nearly everyone agrees with the first sentence. Abortion advocates reject the second sentence. So, that is where more formal pro-life advocacy education begins.

Attacks on humanity

If you've laid a good foundation by showing the Baby Olivia video and intrauterine photos and videos, most young people will recoil from the kinds of dehumanizing arguments abortion advocates advance. But you can show them how Planned Parenthood ignores the presence of the child in the womb when describing abortion; and even when it does refer to the child, it uses dehumanizing language such as "products of conception," "uterine contents," "undifferentiated cell mass," "clump of cells," "pregnancy tissue," etc. Explore these claims and contrast them with what Planned Parenthood formerly taught, that human life begins at conception and that "abortion kills the life of a baby after it has begun."[167] Remind them what they have seen in the videos and ask to hear how they would answer someone who suggests that preborn children aren't human. If preborn children *are* human, and abortion intentionally kills them, then the only conclusion we can draw is that abortion is wrong. Discuss what people should do when they know that an action is wrong, especially when a wrong action leads to the deaths of innocent humans.

Attacks on personhood

You can report that many abortion advocates freely admit that preborn children are, in fact, human beings. They will not, however, admit that children in the womb are "persons" in the same way that post-born people are persons. They want to change the argument you are using as a foundation to say that it's only wrong to kill human beings who count as persons.

The best way to organize this lesson is by using Stephen Schwarz's SLED device.[168] He explains that all the personhood arguments fall into one of four categories: Size, Level of Development, Environment, and Degree of Dependency. You can show that these are terrible standards for determining whether someone should live or die.

We don't say that tall people are more valuable than short people. We don't say that eighteen-year-old women are more valuable than their eight-year-old sisters just because the older females have fully developed reproductive systems while the younger ones do not. No one argues that someone's life or death value comes from where they happen to be located. And we have laws that protect weak and dependent people—so why doesn't that protection extend to smaller, defenseless people in the womb?

The truth is that we are all human persons from the moment of our conception. If all human beings are persons, then The Syllogism holds. Abortion intentionally kills those human persons, which means that abortion is wrong.

You can dive deeper by exploring the reasons given for making the human being/human person distinction. The abortion industry wants to create a class of human beings that it is morally permissible to kill. Philosopher Christopher Kaczor notes that every time this idea has been adopted in all of human history, a moral catastrophe has taken place.[169] Give several examples from history: slavery in the South before the Civil War, or the Armenian genocide in WWI, or the intentional killing of Jews and others the Nazis deemed "defective" in WWII Germany. Discuss why it is critically important to value *all* people.

Hard cases

One of the most emotionally difficult arguments to engage comes up when abortion advocates ask, "What about victims of rape or incest? Are you going to force that woman to give birth to a rapist's child?" You can discuss the standards people use in making these arguments. Primarily, they argue that abortion is warranted in such cases because the woman did not consent to sexual relations and forcing her to give birth to that child would be a constant reminder of the rape. Acknowledge that rape and incest are both horrible crimes and that people who are caught, tried, and convicted of those crimes should be punished to the fullest extent of the law. But the circumstances of someone's conception have no bearing at all on what the one conceived *is*. The child is not the rapist. The child is an innocent third party. Should an innocent third party be killed for the crime of someone else?

As you look at hard case arguments, point out that those who use them have abandoned The Syllogism and are arguing outside of it. You already have demonstrated that abortion is wrong because it intentionally kills an innocent human person. How that child came to be doesn't change the wrongness of intentionally killing them.

The impacts of pregnancy

By far the largest number of pro-abortion arguments regard the impact of pregnancy on the mother. In the lesson outlines available at contendforlife.com/resources, you will engage with the rationale behind each kind of argument in greater detail. Impact-of-pregnancy arguments claim that abortion is necessary because:

- Pregnancy can put at risk the lives of mothers;
- Pregnancy can put at risk the health of mothers;
- Women have the right to do what they want with their own bodies (the "bodily autonomy" argument);
- Pregnancy puts at risk the psychological and economic well-being of the woman;
- Social stigma still attaches to pregnancies out of wedlock;
- The pregnant woman is "too young" or "too old";
- Abnormalities that may occur in the developing child will put strain on the woman;
- The child is not the desired gender;
- The preborn child is "unwanted";
- The planet is overpopulated and can't handle more children.

Instead of grouping all these together and rushing through them, give each argument the consideration it deserves. Always remember to *respectfully* explain the positions of abortion advocates so that it will be clear that you are giving each a fair hearing. Then respond to each argument, explaining its flaws in reasoning. Consider a few examples:

For life-of-the-mother claims, note how no state in the United States forbids a physician from treating a woman with a life-threatening pregnancy. Have them try to find an example of a doctor who has been successfully prosecuted for treating a woman with an ectopic pregnancy. Examine a variety of health complications that sometimes occur during pregnancy—for example, preeclampsia or placenta previa—and learn the standard of care for each. You will find that monitoring the pregnancy, and sometimes early delivery, is the normal recommendation.

Remind your students that these claims, like the "hard cases" arguments before them, land outside of The Syllogism. So, unless they can somehow prove that children in the womb are not human persons, then abortion is still wrong. Talk about the motivation people might have for shifting away from the original argument. Discuss, for example, how focusing on the impact of pregnancy shifts the attention to the woman's experience and away from the human child who is being intentionally killed.

The nature of abortion and what it does

As noted in an earlier chapter on language, abortion advocates go out of their way to obscure the nature of abortion and what it does to the bodies of its targets. Instead, abortion is described as "health care" or "a medical procedure that terminates a pregnancy." Just as video and images of preborn children provide proof that what is in a woman's body after conception is much more than "just a clump of cells," describing and providing images of abortion procedures can overcome any claim that abortion is "health care." Abort73 offers a highly detailed, fully source-cited description of types of abortion procedures, along with a page of images.[170] The Center for Bio-Ethical Reform, on its AbortionNo website, provides both images and videos of actual abortions.[171]

Some question whether using images is necessary, but history demonstrates that photographs, film, and video of human travesty are powerful tools to create natural aversion. Images of lynching, and films and photographs of concentration camps in Nazi Germany, both shocked the conscience of the nation. Imagery led to the prosecution of lynch mobs and hardened the resolve of the U.S. regarding its involvement in WWII.[172] Similarly, knowing the truth about what happens in an abortion, and seeing its results, reveals the nature of abortion as the intentional killing of human persons. Most people can hardly bear to look at abortion. The revulsion produced by actual abortion images indicates that the action so portrayed should never take place. No one should encourage others toward abortion or allow it to remain legal in a just society.

Directly Engaging Pro-Abortion Strategies

As young people approach voting age, help them see their role as citizens in working to end abortion. The next two chapters will explore legislative issues and strategies, and ways the church and pregnancy centers do the important work of changing and shaping worldviews about abortion. Both chapters contain action steps. Anyone willing to honestly assess their gifts, talents, and resources will be able to find something to do and some way to help.

A pro-life worldview should permeate your family and your church, leading to tangible results. Encourage young people to get married and have children, if they can. Everyone in the church should demonstrate love and support for the children of others, even in something as simple as showing kindness to parents whose babies cry during the sermon. Advocate for pregnant teens who want to be a part of church. Visibly partner with your local pregnancy center through regular prayer, donations, and volunteering. *Something* can always be done to connect your family and your church to life-affirming ministries.

Education is the Precursor to Action

For many decades, the silence in the church about the intentional killing of preborn children has opened the door for abortion advocates to fill that vacuum. Those who want to continue abortion command the messaging in virtually every public forum: government, education, medicine, and media. Before the culture can be changed, advocates for life must do the hard work of educating their families, churches, and communities.

You can be a part of that solution.

Unmask the immoral messaging of the abortion industry and replace it with the truth. Share the scientific, moral, and biblical evidence and make a solid case for life. When you get the information out, it will find its way to voters, clarify life issues for them, and reveal the way they should vote and act.

In the next chapter, you will discover public-policy agendas – what works, what doesn't – and how we can move forward with life-affirming laws.

PIVOT 3

DON'T BE COMPLACENT; REINFORCE

CHAPTER 9

Locking Down Policy in Pro-Life States

Prior to 1910, it was legal throughout the United States to pay a woman for sex. Wife beating was first outlawed in the U.S. in the state of Tennessee in 1850, but it took until 1920 before it was criminalized throughout the country. It took many more steps after that to secure voting rights for females. Our nation had to fight a civil war to end chattel slavery, but legally it was finished with the ratification of the 13th amendment to the Constitution in 1865. Dueling was *never* nationally repudiated. It took a march through state legislatures, beginning with Vermont and North Carolina in 1802 and ending with Florida in 1920, for the final state to outlaw the practice.

The Declaration of Independence in 1776 established the rationale for a new nation: "We hold these truths to be self-evident, that all men are created equal, that they are endowed by their Creator with certain unalienable rights, that among these are life, liberty, and the pursuit of happiness. That, to secure these rights, governments are instituted among men, deriving their just powers from the consent of the governed." And yet for decades, that Declaration, along with the Constitution that followed it, allowed prostitution, spousal abuse, dueling, and chattel slavery in the Republic.

But wait! Weren't our founders highly religious? Didn't the majority self-identify as Christian? Research varies and hard numbers are difficult to come by, but in 1800 the vast majority of Americans would have associated themselves with religion. Nearly all children born were baptized.[173] Most believe that these people were far more "religious" than the average American today, something especially true among their leadership.

Compare this perception to the 2026 hard survey data from George Barna and the Cultural Research Center at Arizona Christian University. It reports: "Although the national biblical worldview level among all American adults is only 4%, the levels recorded among younger generations are considerably lower. Among the adult portion of Gen Z (ages 18-22) a mere 1% have a biblical worldview and among Millennials (ages 23-41) that number is 2%."[174]

On one hand, most contemporary people (and certainly most conservative Christians) believe that our nation's founding leaders were largely Christian. On the other hand, based on the kinds of behavior legal at the time, you might judge our forebears as licentious, abusive, violent, and racist. It's hard to hold both ideas simultaneously. I imagine that among our founders who were serious about their faith, we would find agreement that much needed to change in order to produce a truly moral nation.

Didn't our leaders know such things were evil and should not be allowed? Didn't they recognize the dehumanizing foundation of prostitution, wife abuse, and slavery, or the misguided elevation of one man's "honor" over another man's physical life? If so, then why did it take decades, and in some cases more than a century, to legislate relief in response to those problems? Were leaders unwilling? Disinterested? I submit that they didn't fix the problems because they lacked the votes.

Both they and the general populace needed to be educated, persuaded, and exhorted to have unjust ideas driven out and replaced with right thinking. The people needed to elect morally virtuous representatives to pass the necessary laws. Our government requires "the consent of the governed." Once reformers managed to overcome opposition and constitutional hurdles, those who wished to hold on to abusive, rapacious, violent behavior could be compelled by the law to obey. If they did not, they faced the consequences of legal enforcement. In the case of slavery, a bloody civil war preceded legislative relief.

Not Much Has Changed

The country you inhabit today is no different. The "governed" have consented to all manner of horrid behavior. In some states, mind-altering drugs, some of which permanently damage the brains of their users, are legal to purchase and to consume. Euthanasia, another name for the intentional killing of post-born people, is spreading. "No-fault divorce" is wrecking families and pervasive pornography is destroying the ability of young men and women to relate to one another in a healthy way.

Abortion, the intentional killing of innocent children in the womb, continues unabated in many states, while pro-abortion states feel free to violate the laws of pro-life states by sending chemical abortion drugs through the mail. Just because some actions appear inherently unjust, even Constitutionally unsupportable, doesn't mean that those actions are illegal. They exist because appropriate remedies currently reside outside of "the consent of the governed."

Until citizens of this country are educated, persuaded, and exhorted by individuals like you, little hope exists for a national answer to the problem of abortion. Even at the state level, many are so in thrall to the abortion industry that a legislative solution at this time is premature. As noted earlier, education and worldview change come first, legislation after.

Pro-Life States Can Act Now

If you live in a pro-life state, you can do a great deal right now. Just as anti-dueling laws required state-by-state persuasion, and only then legislation, the same approach is required at this point in the battle for the lives of preborn children. If your pro-life state is to be a light in the darkness, a model for other life states to emulate, and a contrast for residents of abortion states to consider, then pro-life states must reinforce and strengthen their current policies.

In this chapter, I will explore eight areas where state legislation can make a difference:

- Moving from gestational limit laws to life protection laws;
- A state-level "Mexico City Policy";
- Expansion of cross-state civil suits;
- Penalizing corporate sponsorship of abortion
- Advertising regulations to prohibit enticing people to commit a felony;
- Reclassifying abortion drugs;
- Requiring science-based pre-natal education and curriculum on state law regarding abortion; and
- Cooperation between state government and pregnancy help organizations.

There is no impenetrable barrier to making such policies a reality in pro-life states.

From Gestational Age Restrictions to Life Protection Acts

As I speak across the country, I pay careful attention to the laws in each state so that I can address its specific needs. I divide states into three categories: death states (those that have enshrined *Roe*-like laws into their state constitutions), gestational age-restrictive states (those with restrictions based on some arbitrary number of weeks of gestation), and life states (preference goes to states with full life-protection laws, but I include "heartbeat bill" states in this category, because these laws virtually ban abortion).

Death states don't have epiphanies. We have no examples of ideologically pro-abortion states flipping straight to a pro-life policy. Since *Dobbs*, ideologically committed abortion states and life states have moved to entrench their positions. Even states such as Arizona, which had on the books an 1864 territorial law outlawing abortion, should have immediately become a life state after *Roe v. Wade* was overturned. Instead, the state passed a constitutional amendment that functionally allows for abortion throughout pregnancy due to "health exceptions." Reliance on a law over a century old could not overcome the will of the people to choose a comprehensive pro-abortion position. Arizona confirmed its death state status.

People claim that they would rush into a burning building to save a child. I assume these same people teach their own children not to play with matches. Surely, then, to save children from an avoidable death, we should be willing to educate our young people against the danger of abortion.

Florida paints a different picture. A 1989 state supreme court ruling established a constitutional right to abortion. It was eventually overturned and in 2022 Florida enacted a fifteen-week gestational limit ban. Finally, in 2023, legislators had the votes for a "heartbeat bill." An attempt to create a state constitutional right to abortion failed in 2024, only because the threshold for passage was sixty percent. Had it been fifty percent, Florida would now be a state with no restrictions on abortion.

I confess up front that I do not like gestational-age arguments because I recognize that they are not grounded in the easily demonstrated truth of science, that life begins at conception. Gestational-age limit laws, while protecting some children from abortion, also create a class of human beings that it is legally permissible to kill.

But I don't always get to argue in contexts that I prefer. At least since *Roe*, Americans have been conditioned to accept gestational-age arguments. Advocates therefore can and should make relational claims ("from the moment of conception, what is in your womb is your child"); but regarding legislation, we must also speak in the language that those who haven't yet encountered a comprehensive case for life can understand and respond to favorably.

The primary task for any death state or gestational age-restrictive state is to do whatever is legislatively possible to "move the needle" toward increasing protection for the lives of preborn children. If a pro-abortion state like California decided to enact a twenty-week restriction on abortion, it would stop only one percent of all abortions (approximately). Yet such a law would create a platform from which abortion could be more easily challenged. It isn't hard to demonstrate the arbitrary nature of a twenty-week ban. Some states have twelve-week restrictions. Florida initially set restrictions at fifteen weeks, then at six weeks. Real-world examples demonstrate that increasing life protection can happen by legislating gestational-age limit bans.

Legislative victories are not always possible in a diverse, often ungodly, democratic republic; but the educational value of the campaigns alone can help shift the attitudes of certain citizens. Each state represents unique challenges and opportunities. The goal is to educate citizens and legislatures so that they will take the next achievable step and protect the lives of as many preborn children as possible. And for states with legislation similar to Tennessee's Human Life Protection Act, there's still much that can be done to solidify that state's commitment to children.

State-level Mexico City Policy

No clearer delineation exists between the two major political parties in the United States than the way each treat what is known as The Mexico City Policy. Enacted via executive order by President Ronald Reagan in

1984, the Mexico City Policy required "foreign nongovernmental organizations receiving USAID family planning assistance to certify that they would not perform or actively promote abortion as a method of family planning, even if such activities were conducted with non-U.S. funds."[175] Since its inception, every time there has been a Republican president, the policy is enforced. Every time a Democrat holds the White House, the policy is rescinded.

Every pro-life state should have a kind of state-level Mexico City Policy achieved through legislation, not through executive order. Some pro-life states have taken certain steps, such as separating Planned Parenthood from their Medicaid program. But I suggest something that goes much deeper, tying directly into the rationale for state pro-life protection laws.

Breaking Up Shouldn't Be Hard to Do

Pro-life protection laws exist in pro-life states because voting-age citizens have determined that intentionally killing an innocent human being in the womb is illegal. Since performing abortions is illegal, why should the state engage with, encourage, or allow organizations that provide or support abortion to exist under a state mandate? As a public policy, ideas are always up for debate, but open support for activity identified in state statute as criminal should be cause for exclusion.

Earlier, I noted that Nevada brothels can't advertise their services in states where prostitution is outlawed; but organizations such as Decriminalize Sex Work are free to try to influence public policy on that topic in other states.[176] What you won't find on the Decriminalize Sex Work website are addresses of prostitutes or bordellos in states where it is legal, or links to organizations that will facilitate travel and services for those interested in purchasing sex.

Debating public policy is protected by the first amendment, but abortion advocacy organizations go far beyond debating abortion as a public policy issue or trying to alter the law. They encourage, promote, and facilitate abortions, regardless of any state's regulations.

A state-level Mexico City Policy would restrict any organization that encourages, provides, or promotes abortion anywhere from any presence in state-funded educational institutions. Some states have successfully done exactly this. Arkansas passed "The Arkansas Student Protection Act" in 2021.[177] Iowa passed a similar law, upheld by the Iowa Supreme Court in 2021. The court's rationale for upholding the ban on Planned Parenthood's involvement in the teaching of sex education could easily be applied to many other intersections between pro-life states and abortion businesses: "The state could also be concerned that using abortion providers to deliver sex education programs to teenage students would create relationships between the abortion provider and the students the state does not wish to foster in light of its policy preference for childbirth over abortion."[178]

Pro-life states should pass and enforce laws that support their "policy preference for childbirth over abortion." States really can have a vested interest in protecting the lives of preborn children over the interest of an abortion industry that wants to intentionally kill them. All pro-life states should act accordingly and aggressively.

Cross-State Civil Suits

Texas's HB 7, signed into law in 2025, allows abortion-injured parties (including a father deprived of his child) to sue for relief.[179] Monetary damages can be as high as $100,000 per complaint. No successful lawsuits have been brought to date, but even the potential for that outcome will likely create a chilling effect, as people considering abortion in Texas weigh the risk of civil litigation accompanied by financial penalties.

Oklahoma went a step further and criminalized the distribution of abortion pills, with penalties up to ten years in prison and a $100,000 fine. I have only one major complaint with the wording of this statute, found in Section 1. D., which reads:

> This act does not apply to a pharmacist or a manufacturer or distributor of drugs or surgical supplies who lawfully manufactures, possesses, offers, sells, or distributes, in the usual course of that entity's business or profession, any drug, medicine, or instrument intended for any lawful medical purpose.[180]

I'm not an attorney, but the wording does not specify the location of "any lawful medical purpose." Abortion states often argue that since the dispensing of abortion drugs is lawful in their states, and because the dispensing takes place within their state, the fact that those drugs may violate the law in another state has no impact on prescription or distribution. I would like to see the wording amended to "any medical purpose that is lawful in the state of Oklahoma."

Shield laws have been, and will be, invoked by abortion states to protect their abortionists from civil, criminal, and other penalties associated with providing chemical abortion drugs, but that can last only so long. With suits or criminal charges coming from Texas, Louisiana, and other states, the federal courts will have to become involved to settle this interstate dispute. In particular, regarding abortion pills, how can abortion states continue to flagrantly violate the law in pro-life states? At the time of this writing, *Louisiana v. FDA* is on appeal to the Supreme Court. The justices will determine whether states may effectively regulate their own borders and so prohibit mail-order abortion pills.

The more pro-life states that pass laws like Texas' HB 7 and Oklahoma's HB 1168, and then move to enforce them, the greater will be the pressure to resolve the controversy. Either the Supreme Court will determine that abortion states have a legal veto over pro-life states, or the majority of the justices will hold that mail cannot be used as a weapon to thwart laws in pro-life states.

Nothing in these state-level, life-affirming laws would stop abortion from continuing in abortion states such as California, New Mexico, and Illinois. Abortion "tourism" would continue. Such laws would, however, draw a more distinct divide between life states and abortion states, which under current law remains blurry. Other approaches might further stem the tide of interstate abortion.

Abortion Trafficking

Over one hundred cities and counties across seven states (primarily in Texas) have passed laws prohibiting abortion. Over fifty of those laws also seek to stop abortion trafficking.[181] These ordinances provide for civil penalties for people who transport pregnant women across the covered territory for the purposes of obtaining abortions, even if those abortions are eventually performed out of state. Anti-trafficking laws have been spearheaded by Mark Lee Dickson, founder of the Sanctuary Cities for the Unborn initiative. He explains that:

> These ordinances: (1) prohibit performing elective abortions and aiding or abetting elective abortions within the jurisdiction of the political subdivision, (2) prohibit elective abortions on residents of the political subdivision—regardless of where the abortion takes place, (3) prohibit abortion trafficking through the political subdivision, (4) prohibit abortion-inducing drugs being mailed or brought into the political subdivision, (5) prohibit criminal organizations from doing business inside the political subdivision, and (6) prohibit the transport and disposal of the remains of unborn children killed by an elective abortion by abortion providers outside of the State of Texas from being brought through or disposed of in the political subdivision.[182]

Some counties, relying on language in the Comstock Act (which makes it illegal to use the mail to send drugs or other materials to perform abortions), could designate as "criminal organizations" groups such as Planned Parenthood, because they are abortion providers and facilitators.[183] As such, abortion businesses, or abortion-adjacent businesses. would be disallowed the right to do any business inside the political subdivision.

Criminal Organizations

Planned Parenthood of Tennessee and North Mississippi could be a case in point. The organization has a section on its website called Patient Navigation Services. The page reveals that the organization knows abortion is banned in both states. So, it created a Patient Navigation team specifically designed to facilitate client abortions in other states while at the same time undermining legitimate pregnancy help organizations (many of whom receive state funding), referring to them as "fake clinics."[184] Why would an in-state, non-profit organization that not only flagrantly encourages citizens in pro-life states to engage in a behavior that would be illegal in that state, but also helps them to navigate the process, be allowed to continue such behavior unopposed? Anti-trafficking ordinances might put a stop to it.

Enforcement of these ordinances happens through private citizen victims, empowered by the law to seek civil damages against anyone found by a court to be in violation. While no civil suits utilizing these ordinances have yet succeeded, their passage provides two immediate benefits. First, they serve as a declaration of the intent of the city or county that initiates them, providing an even firmer foundation for the kind of educational proposals outlined in the previous chapter. Second, they serve as a type of "escape hatch" for girls and women being pressured by others to abort their children. It gives her the chance to respond, "I can't. It's illegal. And you might get sued."

Ending Corporate Sponsorship of Abortion

A simple online search conducted early in 2026 reveals that the grocery chain giant, Kroger, provides up to $4,000 in travel costs to pay for their employees working in pro-life states to intentionally kill their preborn children in abortion states.[185] Kroger has a large corporate footprint in pro-life states.

Over two dozen major companies offer similar travel programs for their employees working in pro-life states who seek to abort their children. Included in that list are companies such as Starbucks, Zillow, Apple, Microsoft, Disney, Netflix, and Dick's Sporting Goods.[186] These companies have a financial incentive to encourage employees to abort.

Female employees who give birth may need maternity leave, take more days off due to child-related issues, and might place children on company health care policies. The mere existence of the offer of $4,000 for an employee to travel to another state to intentionally kill her child telegraphs the company's priorities.

Pro-life states should pass legislation prohibiting employers from financial enticement or assisting ("aiding and abetting") individuals in procuring an abortion. Such laws should stop employers from incentivizing abortion by offering travel funds. While abortion travel fund bans would apply only to those corporate entities and employees located within a pro-life state, it would represent another example of a state legislating in favor of its policy preference that children should be born and not aborted. A pro-life state can't make a national abortion-supporting corporation change its mind, but it can certainly require the company to change its policies that affect the citizens inside its borders.

Such legislation might draw litigation. While some companies might relish the prospect of striking a blow for intentional child killing, many would not. Companies that have a family-friendly brand might hesitate to bring public attention to their corporate financing of abortion. As a result, businesses with branches inside protected locations might simply choose to follow the local ordinance. And while you wait for such legislation, you could choose not to patronize such businesses. But if you do stop shopping with such companies, make sure to write a letter to the local and corporate office telling them why, and what it would take for them to earn your business.

Restrictions on Advertising

While the internet has put regulating abortion advertising beyond the reach of state and local governments, some abortion advocates have taken to traditional advertising to undermine the pro-life protection laws of some states. In an earlier chapter, I noted how Gavin Newsom put up billboards in pro-life states directing readers to the availability of abortion in California. Mayday Health did the same with placards, billboard trucks, and aerial ads.

In *Bigelow v. Virginia* (1975), the Supreme Court upheld the right to advertise abortion across state lines. That was in 1975, just two years following *Roe v. Wade*. Even today, any legal issue that is "abortion-adjacent" will be politically fraught in ways that other issues are not.

In Tennessee, for example, marijuana sales are illegal. The state takes it a step further in the Tennessee Code, which notes, "It is unlawful for any person to place in any newspaper, magazine, handbill, or other publication, any advertisement, knowing, or under circumstances where one reasonably should know, that the purpose of the advertisement, in whole or in part, is to promote the sale of objects designed or intended for use as drug paraphernalia." No one can advertise drug paraphernalia because it is used to facilitate illegal drug use.

If abortion is a crime in your state, then why should out-of-state actors be allowed to advertise a product or procedure designed to intentionally kill children in violation of state law? I can't make sense of the juxtaposition that restrictions on advertising for drug paraphernalia or prostitution in states where both are illegal are acceptable, but restrictions on advertising for abortion are somehow different. Bad legal precedent can be removed only by constitutional amendment or by a later court overturning an earlier court's ruling. Some challenges have already begun.

Tennessee passed related legislation in 2024, known as the "abortion trafficking law," that makes it illegal to "recruit" a minor to procure an abortion in another state. Opponents sued, claiming that the law unconstitutionally restricts free speech. Implementation of the law has been blocked so far by court rulings. At the time of this writing, an appeal of the ruling in the case (*Welty v. Dunaway*) is pending before the Sixth Circuit Court of Appeals. In a post-*Roe* legal environment, if more pro-life states pass laws prohibiting abortion businesses from recruiting or promoting abortion via advertising in their state, it could build pressure and potentially lead to an overturning of *Bigelow*.

South Dakota's success in its litigation against Mayday Health may point to reluctance among abortion supporters to test the precedent.[187] Winning would clear the way for states to protect their youngest citizens from predatory advertising designed to elicit what would constitute felony behavior in that state.

Reclassifying Drugs that May Cause Abortions

Ever have a terrible cold? You might be old enough to remember a time when itchy eyes and a runny nose could be treated by walking into a pharmacy, snatching a package of Sudafed off the shelf, paying the cashier, and walking out. If you are under thirty, that scenario sounds like a fantasy. You know that Sudafed can't be found on the shelves; it's a behind-the-pharmacy-counter drug. You don't need to have a prescription to purchase it, but you do have to provide your driver's license or a government-issued photo ID. That's because in 2005 the federal government passed The Combat Methamphetamine Epidemic Act.

Sudafed contains pseudoephedrine, a key component in the illegal manufacture of meth. Drug dealing outfits used to go in and buy it by the cartful. In an attempt to stem the flood of meth, therefore, the federal government placed limits on who could get it and how much they could purchase, because some people were using this benign cold medication for nefarious purposes.

The two drugs used in chemical abortions, mifepristone and misoprostol, are already prescription medications in the U.S. Like Sudafed, both of these drugs have benign, ethical uses, so they need to be available. But since both can be used in harmful ways they need to be reclassified.

Louisiana is the first state to move mifepristone and misoprostol into Schedule IV of their Uniform Controlled Dangerous Substances Law.[188] Illegal possession of these drugs could lead to fines and jail time. I urge pro-life states to consider the following:

- Place mifepristone and misoprostol on their list of controlled substances;
- Require a negative pregnancy test as a prerequisite for prescriptions for mifepristone and misoprostol;
- Provide for fines and imprisonment for physicians and pharmacies who disregard the negative pregnancy test provision and prescribe these drugs for home use;
- Include penalties for anyone in possession of mifepristone and misoprostol without a valid prescription.

Such legislation would bar any in-state pharmacy from dispensing chemical abortions, while still allowing them to dispense mifepristone or misoprostol for legitimate health reasons. On its own, this wouldn't stop e-tail abortion businesses from shipping pills into pro-life states. But fear of prosecution for illegal possession might stop many, especially men or mothers of pregnant teens, from ordering them. In conjunction with the other approaches in this chapter, it could continue to create the kind of pressure leading to federal action, drawing a more definitive line between life and death states.

Many of the methods discussed above come in the form of restrictions on abortion, abortion methods, or abortion recruitment and trafficking. In other words, they focus on direct abortion actions without doing much to create or advance a culture of life. Pro-life states can signal their support for children, parents, and family formation through public education and life-affirming partnerships.

Enact Life-Affirming Curriculum

It would be absurd for a state to require student drivers to master its traffic laws to protect themselves and others, but be unable to require students to learn about its life-affirming legislation to protect themselves and others.

In the preceding chapter, I laid out the kind of education that parents and churches could provide their children. Some of that curriculum is explicitly "religious" and may face barriers in government-run schools. Nevertheless, there is no reason why pro-life states can't require public schools to teach students the law and provide the underlying scientific and moral rationale for it.

Pro-life states can and should introduce students to pro-abortion laws in other states, such as California, and explain how those laws uphold behavior that violates basic scientific facts regarding the beginning of human life and the nature of preborn children in the womb. Because pro-abortion laws allow for abortion, curriculum should expose students to the violent nature of abortion. Such curriculum should also explore the nature of personhood, in particular how all humans are persons, and explain how the arbitrary definitions of personhood used by states that advocate abortion ideology place *all* human beings at risk.

States may pass laws that reflect their own policy goals; and if a state has determined that its power should protect preborn human life, it has an obligation to teach its young citizens *why*.

Financially Partner with Life-Affirming Agencies—But Beware

If California can spend hundreds of millions of taxpayer dollars to affirm abortion and partner with organizations that intentionally kill children, then pro-life states can do likewise in support of life-affirming organizations. Fortunately, in twenty-one states, including Texas and Tennessee, PHCs already receive varying levels of taxpayer-supported funding. Find out what kind of support is available to PHCs in your state and encourage your state representatives to consider increasing it.

I see something inherently beautiful about life-affirming states that tangibly support life-affirming organizations and pregnancy help centers and clinics. Remember, though, that political winds are fickle. A pro-life state this election cycle can become an abortion-advocating state the next. Enacting the educational policies outlined above will go a long way toward locking the state down for life; but political realities require caution.

Pro-life educational organizations and pregnancy help centers should limit the use of state funding to one-off expenditures, such as ultrasound machines, physical plant, maybe even bulk diaper purchases. Taxpayer money exerts a very strong temptation, but organizations that come to rely on it discover that it arrives with strings. The same hands that gave it can take it away. No organization should risk counting on state grants for ongoing operational expenses in *any* form. Knowing that money is fungible—that using it in a designated area can free up other funds to use elsewhere—should drive you to sequester these funds for one-time uses only.

Always raise critical support privately. Create a "rainy-day" fund. One of the quickest ways for the enemies of life to destroy the life-affirming infrastructure of a state would be to suddenly withdraw funding from those groups who have become dependent on them. Use such funds, but never *ever* rely on them.

Stay Focused

As you can see, there are a host of strategies and tactics pro-life states can employ to strengthen protections for children in the womb. Depending on the commitment level of the electorate, some states can do more, while in other states it may take time to build the necessary consensus to move forward. While it's important to stay focused, it's also necessary to avoid distractions that might derail your progress. In the next chapter, I'll look at one splinter faction whose goal – the end of legal abortion – is shared by every pro-life supporter I know. Unfortunately, their chosen approach isn't difficult, it's impossible, and, because of that, pursuing it dilutes efforts and resources better expended saving the lives of preborn children at risk.

CHAPTER 10

Avoid Distractions That Can't Work

Every pro-lifer I know is an abolitionist; they all want to see an end to elective abortion. But a small sub-section of pro-life people call themselves "Abolitionists." To avoid confusion in this section, I'll use another name that this faction also embraces: Immediatists.

Free The States, an Immediatist website, describes its approach as follows: "Legislatively, we must demand nothing less than the total and immediate abolition of all abortion, or by default we unavoidably give tacit approval to the murder of some."[189]

Incrementalists

People in the Immediatist group frequently use the term "Incrementalist" for pro-lifers who reject Immediatism as an effective strategy. Incrementalists argue that since the immediate abolition of abortion is currently unachievable, everything that *can* be done to save as many lives as possible now *should* be done. Incrementalism as a strategy has to led many victories: gestational limits on abortion, the federal ban on the D&X procedure (commonly known as "partial-birth abortion"), heartbeat bills (some in place even before the overturning of *Roe v. Wade*), the current abortion bans in many states, and even the *Dobbs* decision, all provide examples of positive, incremental movements. Each of these victories came once citizens in a jurisdiction, or the legislators in each governing body, had the votes to achieve them.

Don't let it concern you if any of these terms sound unfamiliar. Unless individuals are already committed and aware actors in the pro-life field, the terms likely would go unrecognized. Despite claims to the contrary by Immediatist groups, my experience in this area of pro-life work tells me that the Immediatist faction is relatively small (though very loud), and I would argue that it doesn't represent a "division" in the pro-life movement as much as a distraction. It has managed to gain some notoriety on TikTok and Facebook Reels. Attempts have been made to get some Immediatist bills considered (though virtually all stall in committee and none have passed). It managed to infiltrate the national Southern Baptist Convention a few years ago which passed a watered-down version of its resolution. Most recently, in 2026, it gained access to the Texas Republican Party convention and got its language adopted among the party's legislative priorities. Both were symbolic victories, at best. SBC member churches are not bound by the resolution and Texas legislators are not required to follow party convention priorities.

But because Immediatists keep raising their voices, primarily in opposition to other pro-life groups, I want to put forward a few key reasons why their approach should be rejected. I will not take an exhaustive look at their claims, however, since this book focuses on outlining the problems posed by the abortion industry's shift in a post-*Roe* world, along with the strategies and tactics that I believe are needed to work toward victory.

Responses to Immediatist Claims

Pro-life apologists such as Gregg Cunningham from the Center for Bio-Ethical Reform and Scott Klusendorf from Life Training Institute have ably debated directly with individuals who have identified themselves as Immediatist leaders (links to both debates, an excellent essay by Craig

Ireland, and a reference to a key chapter in Klusendorf's book are in this endnote).[190] In those debates, both sides present their various biblical, historical, and strategic claims. I submit that Cunningham and Klusendorf won those debates decisively. I encourage you to watch them and come to your own conclusions, but I won't revisit those claims here.

Additionally, arguments regarding whether women are or aren't secondary victims of the abortion industry tend to rely on anecdotal evidence. Immediatists assert that *all* women doubtless know they are killing a human being. Mark Harrington, president of Created Equal, has interacted with countless college students over the years, as has Trevor Polo, executive director of Protect Life Michigan. Additionally, Lincoln Brandenberg has spoken as an apologist to students on innumerable campuses. When I asked all three leaders to assess the understanding of college students regarding the idea that "all human beings are persons" on a scale of 1-10, (1 being lowest), they gave college students failing grades. Harrington ranked them as "3-4."[191] Brandenberg added:

> Generally, "human" is categorized by college students as a stage of development, rather than correctly as a species. When pressed to define when they believe an individual human life begins, they pick points of development that are arbitrary. The baby is largely dehumanized as a "blob." As a former colleague described it: "Pro-abortion student logic is that it's a clump of cells for 9 months, then it suddenly sprouts arms and legs, before popping out!" The concept of personhood is very much separated from the concept of humanity in the minds of modern college students. Even when pro-abortion students concede that the preborn are, by definition, human, the students will often retreat towards the "but it's not a PERSON" philosophical argument.[192]

Myriad interactions with pregnancy help center workers, testimony from women with abortion in their past, and in research I cited earlier regarding the ignorance of college students about fetal development and abortion, demonstrate that while *some* women certainly know that abortion intentionally kills children, many (perhaps most) do not. And even when people admit that preborn children are "human," they don't mean human persons. Instead they create a separate category for children in the womb that makes intentionally killing them, in their minds, morally permissible.

The nation's ignorance is unsurprising, given the decades of state-sponsored propaganda teaching lies about the nature of life in the womb. As noted in the *California Medicine* essay cited earlier, a longstanding campaign has existed, a "schizophrenic sort of subterfuge" designed to "separate the idea of abortion from the idea of killing" and convince people that abortion is factually not the killing of a human being.[193] TikTok posts and Reels of college students continue to amaze me, in which these young adults adamantly proclaim, in campus debates with the late Charlie Kirk and discussions with Mark Harrington of Created Equal, not only the inhumanity of preborn children but even question the status of children in the womb as living beings at all. At best, total moral culpability is elusive. Again, others have ably debated that contention.

The Signature Immediatist Claim

Instead, I want to look at the signature strategic claim advanced by Immediatists: that abortion is murder and therefore the only way to ensure equal protection of preborn children is to pass laws that prosecute, convict for the crime of homicide, and punish the women who abort their children. Immediatist leaders, such as T. Russell Hunter, argue that only Immediatists seek justice, while Incrementalists (representing the overwhelming majority of the pro-life movement, who strive to pass *any* legislation that will result in the saving of as many preborn lives as possible) either do not seek justice or wish to indefinitely delay justice.[194]

To Immediatists, Justice means to tie the intentional killing of preborn children to the 14th Amendment (most Immediatists see that as already the case), thereby declaring abortion legal murder, and then to punish all involved to the fullest extent of the law. Such a legal recognition ideally would take place nationally, but Immediatists have demonstrated a willingness to try to achieve the goal incrementally, on a state-by-state basis. They reject any legislation designed to place limits on intentional child killing and thereby to save lives, instead identifying such laws as "regulating abortion," (rather than what the law actually accomplishes: limiting killing) and therefore unjust. In fact, *all* pro-life people want to see an end to legal abortion. The question is: will a law seeking to prosecute women for the crime of abortion best achieve that goal?

Before I launch into that analysis, I want to clarify what I believe to be a "straw man" argument raised by some in the pro-life movement (even though it is repeated in Hunter's video cited above; a charitable assessment about his meaning is best). Some people say that the Immediatists want to "criminalize women." I don't believe this is the goal. A more accurate assessment is that Immediatists want to universally and immediately criminalize the act of elective abortion, resulting in the prosecution of anyone involved in that act. Still, a substantial emphasis on prosecuting women has been a hallmark of their communication (in the messages I have examined).

Because others named above have looked at the biblical arguments and the historical and legal claims Immediatists advance (you will encounter those in the debates), I want to focus on two claims, one minor and one major. The minor claim is that Immediatists can't pass the legislation they want to advance. The major claim is that, even if they could, the law would be nigh impossible to enforce, leading to undesirable consequences.

No Signs of Success

Some legislation sponsored by Immediatists has made it to committee, and at least once it neared a state house vote; but in no state have Immediatists been able to pass a bill they support. The rationale offered by Immediatists is that the bills *could* pass if establishment pro-life people would get behind them. I'd argue that the bills don't pass because Immediatists can't make compelling arguments for their adoption. Furthermore, I'm not sure why they believe the full support of other pro-life advocates would give them victory, when in many states, pro-lifers can't even pass gestational limit bills or even bare-bones parental notification and consent bills. If Immediatists want wider support, they need to make arguments capable of persuading others, including those who don't share their worldview presuppositions. So far, they haven't managed to draw a critical mass of supporters to their approach in *any* legislative venue. But the problem goes far deeper than legislation.

Even basic pro-life messaging on subjects such as the sanctity of human life, the nature of abortion, fetal development, and the biblical analysis that abortion is modern-day child sacrifice akin to Old Testament Molech worship— topics championed by the pro-life movement for decades—has a very hard time gaining a voice *in most Christian churches* throughout America. Lack of messaging leads to bad outcomes.

When I train pastors, I ask how many of them, in the preceding year, have had a woman seek counseling for an untimely pregnancy or for an abortion in her past. Better than 96 percent say "none." Occasionally one hand will go up; but when I increase the number to "two women," even that hand goes down. Not speaking on the issue creates a vacuum that abortion advocates enthusiastically fill.

Across the U.S., only a small percentage of ministry leaders seek training about how to preach on the sanctity of human life and the dangers of abortion, training I know they desperately need. Many years ago, Barna Group surveys found that only 8 percent of congregants wanted to hear their pastor talk about subjects such as abortion, LGBTQ issues, or same-sex marriage.[195] Barna found that the pressure *not* to speak doesn't come nearly as much from outside the church as from within it.[196] More recently, Barna noted that "only one in five pastors (20%) say they are equipped to lead on 'politics and civic engagement.'"[197] Among response forms completed by pastors who attend my "How to Teach the Toughest Topic" session, many admit they came to the event ignorant in the area of abortion and lacked general equipping to speak confidently about it.

No city, no state, no nation is ever holier than its churches.
You can't expect secular citizens to do the job
the church itself refuses to do.

No city, state, or nation is holier than its churches. You can't expect secular citizens to do the job that the church itself refuses to do. How can anyone think it possible to pass the kind of legislation Immediatists require when more than 40 percent of all abortions are performed on women who were church attenders during the time of the procedure?[198]

Most Americans labor under a worldview that for more than fifty years has taught them to believe a lie. Pro-life advocates have tremendous educational and persuasion hurdles to overcome. Thanks to the tireless efforts of many pro-life organizations and through the model set by the sacrificial work of pregnancy help organizations, some protections are now in place that would have been unimaginable just a few years ago.

"But the number of abortions has gone up since the *Dobbs* decision," goes the common Immediatist reply. What? Did we think that the opponents of life would just lie down? Through their own pivot, they have ramped up chemical abortions and enacted shield laws and are flying death over the ramparts created by life-affirming legislation. Women – who might have been dissuaded from abortion because of the distance between where they live and an abortion facility – now have easy access. That helps to account for an increase. Abortionists managed to expand their target audience and increase market penetration.

Immediatist legislation has demonstrated an inability to pass any laws; but laws such as those enacted in Texas and Louisiana have laid the groundwork to end mail-order abortions in pro-life states, which would represent an incalculable number of lives saved and more firmly divide life states from death states.

The inability of Immediatists to move their legislation forward is the lesser of the two arguments. The major argument says that even if they could get their legislation through, if the law did in fact target women who kill their children in abortion and then seek to prosecute them for homicide, it would be impossible to enforce. Unenforceable legislation gets rejected when it comes before legislators who understand the need for workability, funding, and enforcement.

Unenforceable Laws Are Bad Laws

In response to life-affirming legislation in pro-life states, the abortion industry has pivoted hard to chemical abortions. In chapters three and four, I explored the rapid expansion of this child-killing methodology, showing that abortionists have no qualms about extending it deep into the second trimester and even early into the third trimester. Should they succeed, chemical abortion could make up over 90 percent of all abortions in the U.S.

For those who wish to focus prosecution and punishment on women who intentionally kill children using chemical abortions, four titanic hurdles exist.

1. It's Impossible to Eliminate the Drugs

Senator Josh Hawley introduced a bill in 2026 to remove FDA approval for the use of mifepristone in elective abortions.[199] Depending on the final text of the law, should it secure approval, mifepristone would continue to be used for other purposes, such as treating Cushing's Syndrome or managing miscarriages. The drugs would not go away. In chapter three I describe how a number of states stockpiled the drug because they were fearful of pending legal challenges at the Supreme Court. Any FDA ruling would end up in court.

Even if Hawley's legislation were to be enacted, at least two other routes exist to continue chemical abortions. First, and most likely, is the introduction of alternatives. Ulipristal acetate, commonly known by the brand name Ella, is used for "emergency contraception" and treating uterine fibroids. The preliminary finding of research published in the *New England Journal of Medicine* in 2025 reports that ulipristal acetate works well as an alternative to mifepristone.[200] It is also more widely available and less expensive.

Second, there would be a simple shift to misoprostol-only abortions, as noted in chapter three. Misoprostol was selected as part of the abortion pill protocol because it already was known to cause miscarriage. Misoprostol is used to treat stomach ulcers and in obstetrical procedures that require a ripening of the cervix and induction. When prescribed for such reasons, its warning label cautions women not to use the drug if they are pregnant.

These drugs are here, they aren't going away, alternatives are available and others are being sought. Any drug carrying a risk of miscarriage on the warning label will act like a neon sign to the abortion industry. And as you will see, it is nearly the perfect killing device.

2. Presents Identically to a Miscarriage

One of the greatest challenges to those seeking to prosecute women for abortion is that chemical abortions present identically to natural miscarriage. Approximately 15-20 percent of all known pregnancies end in miscarriage. The number is likely far higher, especially early in pregnancy. Some medical publications suggest the miscarriage rate to be as high as 40 percent of all pregnancies, but many of these miscarriages occur before women know they are pregnant.[201]

One of the complications of chemical abortion is that it sometimes leads to an incomplete abortion. The Maryland-based abortion business, Roxy Clinic, provides this advice to its clients who need to visit urgent care or the ER after an incomplete abortion: "You don't have to tell the provider you took pills. Saying 'I think I'm having a miscarriage' or 'I'm bleeding and I was pregnant' is completely true and leads to exactly the same clinical workup and treatment."[202] And that's not the only way abortion pill abortion is hard to spot.

Imagine the investigative burden. Would state governments be required to investigate every miscarriage to determine whether foul play had taken place? Abortion businesses already advise their clients to claim natural miscarriage, so how will investigators know which ones to pursue? And even if the human resources to investigate were available would the means of ascertaining guilt be possible? Medical research indicates that it is not.

3. Disappearing Drugs

Mifepristone, also known as RU-486, is the first chemical in the abortion pill protocol. Roxy Clinic reports that there are no FDA-approved tests for mifepristone.[203] A recent case study with a single subject demonstrated that mifepristone *could* be detected in a maternal blood test.[204] The subject in the study confessed to abortion pill usage and the blood sample was taken within twenty-four hours of the completion of the abortion. No studies exist to show that mifepristone could be detected later. And if such a test were ever made readily available, the abortion industry has already demonstrated its willingness to substitute other drugs for mifepristone, or forego it altogether and promote misoprostol-only abortions.

Misoprostol, the second of the drugs used in a chemical abortion, can't be detected by a blood test five minutes after it has been taken.[205] The body breaks it down into misoprostol acid, which can't be detected two days after dosage "due to progressive metabolism and/or degradation processes."[206] Back in 2014, the abortion advocacy group Gynuity Health Projects reported that few of these kinds of blood tests are available, even fewer for commercial use, and they are very expensive.[207] Nothing has changed.

The instruments used in the latest published research—ultra-high-performance liquid chromatographs—are expensive, require costly upkeep, and need highly-trained specialists to do the work.[208] The only successful research analysis, involving a total of two cases, required tissue from the body of the fetus or the placenta, neither of which is generally available in a chemical abortion, as both are routinely flushed down the toilet.[209] Even in the instance of an incomplete abortion, routine testing of fetal tissue would not find it; and the kind of testing outlined in the example, especially in cases where there is no immediate accusation of illegal activity, is not done. Even if it were possible (and it's not), it would be exceedingly difficult to fund.

4. Playing 'Hide the Abortionist'

Enforcement roadblocks continue to multiply. AB 260 was signed into law by California Governor Gavin Newsom on October 3, 2025. The bill allows abortion pills to be sent without designating who prescribed the pills or the name or address of the dispensing pharmacy. The law also withholds the name of the patient on the bottle's label. All of this came directly in response to the concern that pro-life states would use such information against abortion businesses operating in shield law-protected abortion states. Teresa Burton, writing for *Ms.*, openly admits the rationale:

> Currently, one in four abortions is obtained via telehealth, half of which are in states with abortion bans or harsh restrictions. Identifying patients, pharmacies and prescribers in order to criminally prosecute or civilly sue them has become central in the conflict

> between states with abortion providers and states with abortion bans. AB 260 is a response to high-profile attempts by conservative states targeting providers of telehealth abortion and their patients. Several states have shield laws to protect patients and prescribers, but arguably no other state law is as comprehensive as California's new confidentiality provisions.[210]

Other abortion states have some privacy provisions; but I expect that all abortion states will quickly use the California law as their model. They purposefully obscure medical information for political purposes. Such measures would further complicate the enforceability of the kinds of state laws Immediatists insist upon.

Unfortunate Consequences of Immediatist Laws

The drugs used in chemical abortion are here to stay because they have legitimate uses in other areas. The effects of chemical abortion are generally indistinguishable from natural miscarriage. And the drugs are impossible (or at best exceedingly difficult) to detect because the means to do so are rare and the investigative burden would be excessive, even intolerable to women. Imagine the response of a grieving, innocent woman, suffering the loss of her baby through natural miscarriage, who has been told that she and/or her stillborn child must now be subject to forensic investigation.

Immediatist laws not only can't be passed, but if they somehow were passed, they couldn't be enforced. While I think it virtually impossible that Immediatist legislation will ever pass, if it were passed, I'd like to explore two very negative unintended consequences.

What About Targeting the Professional Abortion Industry?

The next, most achievable step toward making abortion effectively illegal involves targeting for prosecution those most responsible: professional abortionists and their allies. E-tail abortion and shield laws are a significant reason why abortion numbers continue to climb in the *Dobbs* era. But as states move to close loopholes and attorneys general and district attorneys grow bolder, indictments and lawsuits will come.

I had a conversation at a conference in 2024 with Thomas Glessner, the president of the National Institute of Family and Life Advocates. He advanced yet another key reason why targeting women for prosecution was unwise. Prosecutors need witnesses to convict abortionists. Women and men who have participated in abortion will be reluctant to come forward if they believe they will be prosecuted, certainly so if the penalty they might receive would be death. Some might argue that prosecutors extend immunity all the time to people who commit crimes so they can capture higher-level perpetrators. But the first time a woman is convicted of murder for killing her child and is sentenced to death, how many other women will come forward as witnesses against the abortionist? Perhaps she is the fifth witness who has come forth against the abortionist, but the prosecutor only needs four; so no immunity is extended and handcuffs await. Who would risk it?

An additional consequence: more babies will die. I have met women who took mifepristone and then regretted it. In a perverse way, chemical abortions open a window that surgical abortions do not, namely, a pause between taking the first and second drug. During that interval an intervention can take place.

Since mifepristone by itself is an abortifacient, any woman who might have come forward for Abortion Pill Reversal (APR) treatment, would not do so under Immediatist legislation. The very PHCs that administer the progesterone are also "mandated reporters." They are legally required to report those who abuse or kill children. Knowing a woman has taken mifepristone would trigger a report. APR would vanish and those babies would die, because the fear of prosecution would overcome the shame and regret.

Going after abortionists in civil and criminal court requires willing, able witnesses. If the new ordinances and laws—anti-trafficking, criminalizing e-tail abortion, etc.—are to bear fruit, we must have a laser-beam focus on the chief perpetrators in the abortion industry.

The Problem of Unenforceable Laws Generally

Do you always drive the posted speed limit? I suppose a tiny number of people reading this book would answer "yes," but probably that doesn't describe you. If you're like most people, you not only have exceeded the posted speed limit, but you do so fairly often. You speed because you've done a cost/benefit analysis in your head. You weigh the relatively negligible chance of being caught and fined against whatever reason you have for exceeding the limit. I guarantee that you would never speed if every morning when you pulled out of your driveway, a police cruiser slipped in behind you and followed you to your every destination. But that will never happen. Why not? The U.S. has determined that the resources aren't possible to deploy, even though speeding is a factor in the deaths of nearly 12,000 people nationally every year.

In Maryland, adultery is a misdemeanor crime with a fine of $10. I doubt it surprises you to learn that there have been zero arrests and no convictions in modern times. It's hard to prosecute adultery because it tends to happen in private; both the perpetrator and the victim are likely embarrassed (or, conversely, don't care). Regarding adultery, the U.S. doesn't possess a morality police force, like the one in Iran. Yet the anti-adultery law is still on the books. Does this law act as a tutor? Yes. It teaches people that they can violate some laws with impunity. It would be better if there were no law, than a law everyone feels free to ignore.

Unenforceable laws arise when insufficient resources exist to prosecute violators, when prosecutorial discretion limits prosecution, or in circumstances where it is impossible to successfully prosecute a crime. In the case of abortion, particularly in the era of e-tail and chemical abortion, all three elements are at work. Where will the resources come from to scrutinize miscarriages or to fund and run expensive forensic assays? In many states, prosecutors turn a blind eye and/or judges dismiss cases (or assign probation or exceedingly light sentences) for crimes or perpetrators deemed not worth prosecuting. How might that play out in very liberal jurisdictions (even if they are located in conservative states) that attempt to prosecute, or possibly execute, individual women for abortion?

In the interest of not encouraging drug use, I won't list illegal drugs that are virtually impossible to detect. If not for secondary symptoms, such as driving under the influence, none of the users could be prosecuted. But when chemical abortion drugs are quickly metabolized and leave the body; when misoprostol-only abortions present exactly like spontaneous abortions (miscarriage); how will prosecutions proceed? All states have limited resources to apprehend, try, convict, sentence, and punish those who violate the law. When states don't enforce the law, people feel free to violate the law. Unenforceable laws breed lawlessness.

We must abandon demands to pass unenforceable abortion laws. Pursuing this quixotic quest diverts mental energy, time, and scarce resources that could be devoted to saving the lives of more preborn children now.

Doing What Can Be Done

Until the cultural worldview of most Americans substantially shifts, the goal of making abortion unthinkable and illegal nationwide is far off. Solutions must begin in the church and the home. We will find success most likely first among those who share moral and biblical assumptions about the nature of the preborn and the reality of abortion as the shedding of innocent blood.

It needn't take long, but it absolutely requires will. The greatest obstacle to the advancement of a pro-life worldview is complacency and disinterest.

Mobilizing the church will require an initial appeal to significance. Until Christian people recognize the problem—abortion has been referred to as "the silent subject"—no impetus will exist to find solutions.

I've outlined a few legislative initiatives that I believe are possible to achieve. They either already are present in some pro-life states or they are pending (I hope cross-border e-tail abortion violations will end in successful legal outcomes). Unlike abortion states, most of which operate in near messaging lockstep, pro-life states (and I might add many pro-life organizations) do not.

The unforced errors that plague pro-life organizations and states are partially responsible for creating the environment that prompts Immediatist frustration. But giving in to legislative impulses that can't pass and are impossible to enforce will distract those with workable projects and set back viable achievements. If you are a part of a pro-life organization committed to saving the lives of all of the preborn children that you can, then keep your eyes focused on your goals, work your strategy, and evaluate your outcomes.

The goal is to save as many children at risk from abortion as possible, regardless of differing opinions about the most effective strategy to achieve pro-life goals. Don't sacrifice children in the womb whom you could save right now over the hope of a total ban at some point in the indeterminate future (if it ever comes).

If individuals in pro-life states take the initiative, freely borrow from successful legislation already working in other states, and work together, substantial progress can be made. In the next chapter, I will challenge you to take your role and play your part in one or more of the changes needed to move the battle for life into its next stage – crossing into abortion states to win them for life.

PIVOT

4

DON'T BE FEARFUL; ADVANCE

CHAPTER 11

Breaching Abortion State Walls and Establishing a Beachhead

The Iron Curtain separated the free nations of western Europe from those in the east, who lived under the boot of the Soviet Union. The Mason-Dixon Line in the United States demarked the border between free states and slave states prior to the Civil War.

But the U.S. has resisted any effort to clearly delineate between life states and death states, with designations muddied by the trafficking of chemical abortion drugs from the latter into the former. If, however, life states succeed in implementing the strategies and policies outlined in the previous chapter, the line separating states that protect the lives of preborn children from states that champion their destruction will become increasingly clear.

Unlike the times just before WWII or the Civil War, these sides are not divided by a contiguous land mass. Instead, life states and death states are designated by ideology and policy. Many pro-life states are located in the South and Midwest, but pro-life Idaho is surrounded by abortion states, and until very recently, pro-abortion Illinois was almost completely surrounded by pro-life states. Abortion forces in Missouri flipped the state in 2024 through a constitutional amendment, but an enthusiastic effort to repeal that amendment will appear on the ballot in the fall of 2026.

Do you believe that human life is precious, that children are valuable image-bearers of God from the moment of conception? If so, then the last thing you want is the permanent hardening of dividing lines between abortion states and life states. It is unacceptable to think, "Well, at least *our* kids are safe."

The previous two chapters focused on confirming life states, reinforcing their laws and communicating the rationale for them. But what if you live in, or have friends who reside in, an abortion state? In a state like California, where there appears to be little hope anytime soon for legislation that would provide even meager protections for preborn children, how is it possible that a life ethic could prevail?

Every state can be won for life. Never believe that just because abortion ideology prevails in some states today that it will do so always. It won't. Abortion ideology, and the policies that come from it, are built on lies. The truth absolutely can prevail—but in order to do that, it must be deployed, which means a battle. If you underestimate the resolve of abortion advocates, go back and read the first four chapters. Here, I'll examine the recent conflict in hostile states and why life advocates fared poorly, unpack some reasons for optimism, and describe the beachheads already established.

The Ground Right Now

As abortion states witnessed the forward march of pro-life protection laws, they began to suspect that *Roe v. Wade* was likely to be overturned. They started to entrench their position, working to make the practice of abortion difficult to dislodge.

2024 was a dismal year for pro-life protection laws, with only a few encouraging notes. In South Dakota, citizens beat back a constitutional amendment that would have enshrined the *Roe v. Wade* "trimester" scheme into the state constitution. Florida rejected an amendment that would have made it impossible to pass life-affirming laws or restrictions on abortion. Nebraska passed a lesser measure, placing its twelve-week gestational age restriction into the state constitution (although it still allows over ninety percent of all abortions).

But Arizona, Colorado, Maryland, and Montana all passed constitutional amendments or ballot measures that legalized abortion. Even Missouri, which had banned abortion, passed a constitutional amendment to legalize abortion throughout pregnancy (due to late-term loopholes allowing for abortion if the pregnancy is deemed harmful to a woman's "health," so loosely defined as to be meaningless). New York, already an abortion state, added "pregnancy outcomes" to a list of legally-protected conditions. Nevada, which allowed abortion up to twenty-four weeks gestation (meaning that virtually all abortions are legal there), doubled down with Question 6, a constitutional amendment that would expand legal abortion throughout pregnancy. Question 6 passed on the first vote but is up for a second, confirming vote in the fall of 2026.

In many states where the battle for life was more contentious, abortion supporters outmaneuvered their pro-life opponents. One successful strategy was to combine pro-abortion legislation with other left-leaning, progressive ballot initiatives so as to build coalitions and drive confederates to the polls. In 2024, abortion forces concluded rightly that opportunities to legalize marijuana (Ohio) or creating a constitutional protection for same-sex marriage (Colorado, in case *Obergefell* is overturned) would bring to the polls people who would also favor enshrining abortion rights. Appeals to bodily autonomy can take different forms so that one catalyzes the other at the ballot box.

The language of the pro-abortion initiatives was often purposefully obscure, with the campaigns in favor filled with claims that were untrue. In Missouri, the campaign language for the ballot initiative to amend the constitution to allow for abortion on demand used vague "reproductive rights" language. In Ohio, Rhiannon Carnes, with Ohioans United for Reproductive Rights, represents the typical rhetorical approach of abortion advocates: "Ohioans know that if we don't succeed, the government will have the power to ban abortion completely, even in cases of rape, incest, or when someone's life is in danger."[211] These appeals, right out of Facebook memes appearing after the *Dobbs* decision, claimed that women would be at risk from ectopic pregnancies or couldn't be helped if they miscarried; both were lumped into the category under "abortion." Abortion advocates also repeated the lie that no late-term abortions exist, but if they do, they are rare and always done because of fatal fetal anomaly (more on that false claim below).[212]

Pro-life advocates were caught flat-footed and made strategic errors. Instead of identifying what the ballot measure would do and so ask voters to reject it on principle (difficult, because voters would need to be taught those principles), campaigners thought that appealing to the status quo would win the day. They couldn't have been more wrong.

The Strategic Error

In state after state, the key messaging from the pro-life campaigns declared that the constitutional amendment proposed to codify abortion was "unnecessary and extreme." In Nevada, for example, it argued that the Question 6 constitutional amendment was unnecessary because Nevada already had legal abortion, so the amendment or initiative didn't change anything substantial. Voting "no," then, would keep abortion at the current level. Some pro-life advocates even pointed to current law as making abortion "happen in the safest way possible."[213] In other instances, the new law was labeled as "too extreme" because in many cases the language of the law would allow "abortion up until childbirth." While the claim was completely true in many cases, abortion advocates denied it or minimized its impact.

As anyone can see from the results, these pro-life strategies failed catastrophically.

Why did these arguments fail? Because they didn't give voters a clear alternative, they were subject to being reframed, and it was easy to make them appear implausible.

Enough Abortion

By telling voters that that the new initiative was unnecessary, voters might conclude that the opposing position cared primarily about the threat posed by expanding abortion, but not so much about abortion itself. In other words, it suggested that the amount of abortion the state already had was sufficient, making any new law superfluous.

The status quo positioning of such a communication strategy did nothing to exhort those who might reside in the mushy middle on the issue. So, while committed abortion supporters came out, non-committal voters who may have leaned pro-life didn't see enough advantage and thus sat out.

Abortion Advocates: When There's Doubt, Spread Lies

The minute the *Dobbs* decision leaked, campaigns created to expand abortion used the fabrications already disseminated widely on social media. They made voters feel that if they didn't get behind the push to make abortion a constitutional right, characters right out of *The Handmaid's Tale* would come for their contraception, ban all abortions (including for ectopic pregnancy), women would die from untreated miscarriage, etc.

No state prohibits doctors from treating women with ectopic pregnancies. No physician has ever been successfully prosecuted for aiding a woman with a miscarriage. No legislation exists anywhere in the U.S. that puts access to contraceptives at risk.[214] But telling people, "Oh, that won't happen," after voters already had swallowed the fear-filled narrative was too little, too late.

Make the Truth Unbelievable

One of the most disappointing losses came through pro-abortion campaign language that took something that was true and made it look like a fairy tale. In fact, in many cases these constitutional amendments removed *any* gestational-age restrictions on abortion. So, even if it could be proven that abortions were indeed happening moments before birth, nothing in the law would *prevent* them from happening. The word then went out that the boogeyman of "late-term abortion" was a pro-life scare tactic, it wasn't occurring, and if late-term abortions were happening, it was only on children who couldn't survive long after birth or to save a woman's life.

> Abortion ideology is not restricted by gestational age; it is a worldview committed to 'freedom,' even if that libertine impulse must be purchased with the blood of children.

While it is true that late-term abortions are relatively rare compared to all other abortions—abortions at or after twenty-one weeks make up 1.1 percent of abortions (as noted in chapter three, the earliest verified live birth where the child developed without significant complication after time in a NICU was at 21 weeks' gestation)[215]—removal of all gestational-age restrictions still represent approximately 12,100 dead children. That's no small number.

There is *no* instance in which late-term abortion is necessary to protect the health of the mother. Feel free to search for treatments for all manner of pregnancy complications; you will find that monitoring and early delivery are the recommended approaches. Just because a child may have a birth defect is no reason why the child should be intentionally killed.

Abortion advocates in their campaigns assert that even if there are late-term abortions, they are performed only on children with diagnoses incompatible with life; anencephaly (in which a neural-tube defect causes the cerebrum not to form), for example. But notorious late-term abortionist

Warren Hern admitted to doing abortions up to thirty-two weeks; over half of the children he killed were completely healthy.[216]

Failure to prepare voters far in advance leaves them open to the deceptive claims of abortion advocates. In an election cycle, voters have only a short period in which to make a decision. When the choice they have is between believing an emotionally-compelling bumper-sticker-length narrative (even if false) or working their way through more complex arguments and evidence, the quicker, more dramatic strategy tends to prevail. This is particularly true when individuals are predisposed to believe the lie because it serves their self-interest or salves their conscience.

Even in states most would identify as pro-life, such as Missouri, it was short-sighted to believe that former allegiances would hold, absent ideological reinforcement. As a result, at the time of this writing, Missouri has enshrined abortion on demand as a constitutional right. Having a pro-life "sentiment" is not the same as holding to a pro-life position, undergirded by evidence and reasoning. The pro-life campaign there tried to Get Out The Vote but didn't adequately Get In The Voter. While it's easy to blame the campaign staff, the fact is that the time to Get In The Voter is during worldview creation, not during a political cycle. If people are grounded in the truth, the existence of a campaign to do evil will not persuade them. They'll know the counterfeit when they see it.

Reasons for Optimism

I don't want anyone, especially you, to devolve into "the last angry Christian." That's my term for a New Testament incarnation of Elijah's lament after the wicked Queen Jezebel started chasing him through the desert. "I have been very zealous for the Lord, the God of armies; for the sons of Israel have abandoned Your covenant, torn down Your altars, and killed Your prophets with the sword," Elijah said. "And I alone am left; and they have sought to take my life."[217] The temptation is to think 1) you are the only one left in the battle; and 2) all your most intimidating, powerful enemies are arrayed against you.

Instead, recognize that you have an immeasurable host of like-minded people, many of them fellow Christ-followers, who are just waiting for the instruction and exhortation to jump into the fray. Beyond that are established pro-life organizations waiting to help you. Many have been involved in making educational, legislative, and ministry advances possible, and they are highly motivated to share with you what they know.

Even when circumstances seem difficult and the way ahead virtually impossible, I want to encourage you (no matter what type of state you live in) to become a happy warrior. Not everything is as bleak as abortion advocates would have you believe!

The Myth of Settled Law

A favorite strategy among pro-abortion politicians trying to stave off a change in policy is to talk about "settled law." Over and over again, prior to the *Dobbs* decision, abortion as a "constitutional right" was described as "settled law." And I suppose it was . . . until it wasn't.

The rule of law in the U.S. is *always* subject to "the consent of the governed." When that consent shifts, the prospect for a change in the law becomes possible. It can happen through new referenda, legislation, court rulings, or state or national constitutional amendments.

In other words, don't be cowed by abortion advocates in death states who say things such as "pro-life zealots aren't welcome here," as if the abortion industry owns your state. They might seem to right now, but that doesn't mean that they will tomorrow. Victories, in some cases of limited scope now and statewide and nationwide tomorrow, are always possible.

Despite the Law, Abortion Can Be Stopped

No law in any pro-abortion state *requires* abortion. Abortion is an action that can be stopped. If life-affirming people change the way they talk about intentional child-killing, move to educate others and demonstrate the effectiveness of life-affirming policies in the states where they exist, pro-life advocates won't merely win a debate for "our team." They will save children's lives from those hellbent on destroying them.

The battle is fought with words and votes, but what is at stake are the actual bodies of defenseless humans at risk from abortion. And the best news is that pro-life culture has already made solid inroads into abortion states.

PHCs: The Established Beachhead in Abortion States

Arguments, debates, discussions, and the crafting of points represent the bulk of most books about abortion, including this one. J. Budziszewski, a professor at UT Austin, offers an extension (if not an alternative) of how best to make a case. As he evolved as a persuader, he identified three phases of argument.

In the first phase, the goal is simply to make a better argument. Then you use it, if possible, to help deceived people change their minds.

The second phase involves repeating the incorrect facts and bad reasoning people hold and asking whether the person holding those views really believes them. You might ask, "Right now, are you truly in doubt about the human nature of the fetus in the womb of a human mother?" When pressed, most people will concede the point.

Both phases have an important place in helping others to see the truth about the pro-life position. And they set up the third phase.

While Budziszewski's third phase is often neglected, it is critically important. He describes it this way: "We can meet lunacies not just with counterarguments, but with sounder, more beautiful visions of how things really are. Just having the courage to describe these beauties can be transformative. It can even happen that, at last, at the very last, the longing for beauty overcomes the fear of it."[218]

The Superior Value of PHCs

In the pro-life movement, Budziszewski's third-phase argument is best embodied in pregnancy help centers and clinics. The distinction between Planned Parenthood and PHCs could not be more stark.

Whether women enter Planned Parenthood scared or confident, the true nature of the child in the womb will be hidden from them. If an ultrasound is performed to determine how far along the mother is, the screen will be turned away from her. The Doppler allowing her to hear her baby's heartbeat will be turned off. During any discussion, the presence of the child will be ignored and the child herself dehumanized.

Women entering PHCs may arrive scared and unsure, but they will get honest counsel and often an ultrasound exam revealing the truth about the nature of their preborn children. A new mother will likely receive her very first photo of her child to take home with her and hear her baby's heartbeat.

Mothers visiting Planned Parenthood will spend very little time there. In minutes, or at most over a few days, their children will be dismembered and removed from their wombs while the women are sedated. Alternatively, mothers may deliver their tiny children at home, flushing their children's bodies down the toilet.

Mothers visiting a PHC will get access to classes on everything from childbirth to parenting to job preparation. Perhaps seven months later, these women will go into labor and deliver their beautiful children into the world. Mothers will hold, comfort, feed, and play with their own living miracles, and look lovingly at their children while they safely sleep.

Abortion businesses feed off a mother's desperation and despair, offering her death for her child in exchange for some money and a vague but false promise that her decision is in her own best interest. But intentionally killing your own child is never a positive good, and many women go on to regret their actions.

Pregnancy centers and clinics offer hope and life. Their services are free of charge for the mothers who become clients, and many leave with a new perspective on family formation. Her own life has changed, her priorities as well, and this is a good that will last. The lengths some centers go to sometimes astonish me.

Two Stories

Mariah grew up in a home with an alcoholic father. Her mother passed away when she was twelve. Her experiences took a toll on her, as she fell into addiction and spent time in the sex trade.

She was raising two sets of twins when she became pregnant with a third set. When she couldn't see a way forward, she went to an abortion facility where an abortionist ended their lives.

Later, she discovered she was pregnant again. "I thought if it is twins again, I am getting an abortion."[219] Instead, she walked through the doors of the Pregnancy Resource Center of Rolla in Missouri.[220]

Beset by many fears and challenges, Mariah didn't know how she could take care of six children. Everyday concerns pressed down on her. How would she transport them? "Do they even make eight-passenger cars?" she asked her counselor at the center.[221] Her own vehicle was on its last legs. It's hard for many people to imagine the level of practical desperation felt by many pregnant women.

But the center was on mission, ready to help. It began a GoFundMe account to raise money for a larger car. Before reaching that goal, a local car dealership stepped in and donated an eight-passenger vehicle for Mariah's growing family. The car dealer insisted that he be the one to shoulder this burden, telling the center's CEO, Joe Dalton, "I have been in the car business a long time, but I've only been a Christian for a few months. If anybody can do this, it's me. If anyone should do this, it's me. Please, let me find them a car."[222]

Mariah later earned college degrees in Human Services and Criminal Justice. Today she works hard in her field, alongside the father of the new twins, to support their family.

The abortion industry would look at Mariah's problems as terrible suffering to be avoided through abortion. PRC Rolla saw Mariah's difficulties as opportunities to serve and her children as valuable lives to save.

Kimberly was a client at Bakersfield Pregnancy Center in California. At twenty-three weeks into her pregnancy, a car hit her and she found herself in a wheelchair, needing surgery.[223] Her baby boy, Ryder, was born via C-section; but when his lungs wouldn't clear, he was life-flighted to Valley Children's Hospital in Madera. Bakersfield Pregnancy Center executive director, Erin Rogers, called the pregnancy center in Madera to see if they could help Kim with food, transportation, and hotel accommodations while she was there with her baby. Rogers reports, "Of course, they came through and showed her abundant love and support. It is what the body of Christ does best."[224]

Every day across the country, the staff and supporters of PHCs step into agonizing struggles, remove barriers, and help clients see a path forward for themselves and their children. In other cases, they help clients find forgiveness, healing, and restoration, replacing with hope the emptiness left by a past abortion.

In the battle ahead, PHCs are one of the best physical manifestations of the advantages of embracing a life-affirming worldview. Approximately 2,700 PHCs operate in the United States. Every woman whose child is saved, every man who holds a baby otherwise slated for destruction, all of the grandparents, aunts, uncles and cousins who are positively impacted, are fertile ground for the creation of voices for change. They represent the "beautiful vision of how things really are."[225]

So, what does all that mean for those living in abortion states?

We Need More Centers

Back in the late 1980s, approximately 2,600 abortion facilities existed in the U.S.[226] By 2025, that number dropped to 753 bricks-and-mortar abortion facilities.[227] By contrast, as just noted, approximately 2,700 PHCs operate in the U.S. today.[228] With a nearly four-to-one advantage, why are more PHCs needed?

The raw math can mislead. While it's true that the number of physical abortion facilities has dwindled, many of them relocated from pro-life states that passed pro-life protection laws to more abortion-friendly states. But the number of abortions is rising. It used to be that for a pregnant woman to procure an abortion, she had to visit an abortion facility. Today, she merely needs to open her mailbox. And the United States Postal Service provides more than 170 million points of delivery.[229]

Abortionists have an advantage: a few quick clicks, gather some information, and in minutes the drugs for a chemical abortion can be mailed directly to anyone. The abortion can be completed within a couple of days, with no in-person visit required.

PHCs have worked hard to adapt. Many of their websites now include 24/7/365 Nurse Chat, which enables clients to connect in minutes with a medical professional from their computer, phone, or tablet. But providing pregnancy tests, ultrasounds, counseling, classes, maternity clothes, baby clothes, diapers, wipes, and other physical, emotional, and spiritual support is neither quick nor easy. The work requires a more widespread network of physical PHCs. That is where women, whether brave enough on their own or sufficiently encouraged, can walk through the doors to experience life-changing care.

Abortion lures in women with the quick and seemingly simple promise that they can take some "medicine," their pregnancy will go away, and they can get on with their lives. In reality, they offer human pesticides, their child is intentionally killed, and many women bear the burden of this "solution" for the rest of their lives. PHCs, on the other hand, take the long view.

A baby developing in her mother's womb isn't an "event," but a "process." From a confirmed pregnancy test until birth, seven to eight months go by. During that time, through counseling and mentoring, many women who walked in determined to abort, learn instead to love and bond with their developing child. They discover how to make new and better plans for the future, for both of them. Studying, interacting with mentors through childbirth classes, they prepare themselves and their homes to receive the new baby.

Pregnancy center staff are honest with their clients. Having and raising a baby isn't easy—what of true value ever is?—but it is both rewarding and beautiful.

PHCs as Messaging Hubs

Pastors, lay Christians, and the vast majority of Americans are ignorant about abortion, fetal development, and life issues generally. While many PHCs offer classes to their clients, they are sorely underused as a life messaging hub in their communities. Though centers often have some kind of relationship with area churches, most pastors have never stepped inside a center or clinic, met the director, or taken advantage of the wealth of experience and educational materials PHCs would enthusiastically make available.

How can centers bridge this ministry and educational gap? Through a particular kind of volunteer and by adding a new category of staff.

Church Liaisons

Most PHCs have "church liaisons," sometimes known as ambassadors or facilitators. The job of liaisons is to be the voice of the center to their church, and the voice of the church back to their center. Each church in a service area should have a liaison who meets monthly with executive staff. When programs or curricula become available, churches are informed. When churches, youth groups, or Sunday School classes need a speaker, the liaison can facilitate.

Staff Apologists

In the last few years, I have recommended that pregnancy centers add a new professional position: staff apologist. If that title sounds too intimidating, you could call them Director of Community Engagement (or Outreach). The fact is that the job is too big for most directors to take on. In conversation with a director last year, I asked how many churches were in the center's service area. The answer: about 600. You do the math. If such a director tried to speak just once a week at an area church, it would take more than a decade to get to them all.

But a staff apologist could speak multiple times per week, and not just to full congregations (where it might be tough to get a pastor to give up the pulpit), but to youth groups, small groups, and Sunday School classes. A well-trained apologist could form a speakers bureau made up of staff and volunteers. Instead of waiting for invitations to arrive, they could seek out opportunities to share their message, and not only in churches, but at schools and civic organizations. Imagine how much more could be done if the bulk of the speaking obligations fell on a staff member trained to get those engagements and fill them. Directors would then be free to focus on client services, training, and other executive tasks.

More Ways Forward

Already, in pro-abortion states across the country, there are beachheads of pro-life resistance. In the next chapter, you'll see a number of other strategies being employed so that a pro-life advance can successfully cross borders into hostile territory. But for now, know that the existence and expansion of PHCs is essential. They are the tip of the spear.

CHAPTER 12

Multiplying Voices and Changing Hearts in Hostile States

Fire bombing, spray paint, and threats are the least of it. Open attacks by abortion-supporting state governments fuel individual animosity. As noted in the first part of this book, PHCs are under attack in abortion states. While they bravely hold their ground, if victory is to be achieved, they need lots of help. It must first arrive from the church, but, once properly exhorted, convicted believers will find additional methods to multiply the pro-life voice in hostile states.

From the Church...

Smart center directors, educated pastors, and competent apologists can establish a life-affirming worldview in the local church that can spill out into the community, even in an abortion state. Absolutely nothing stands in the way of grounding Christians in the truth . . . other than a lack of courage.

I wrote *Contenders* specifically for people who message in the church. It helps readers understand how abortion advocates argue in retreat and how to manage the life message. Because I have an extensive background in teaching public speaking, I show how to tailor a message for each audience and each goal, providing different organizational structures to fit the need. I don't have space to repeat all that information here, but it's already available. Go out and get *Contenders.*

Is there a dire need to teach the truth to people in churches located in pro-life states, where Planned Parenthood has been barred from connecting with kids in schools? Yes. So imagine the significance of making inroads into the thought lives of our people languishing in abortion states. Don't forget that forty percent of women who've had abortions were attending church around the same time. That single statistic tells me that the church is a microcosm of the wider community. If the church can't get it right here, it's unlikely to make inroads into the secular culture.

Be Willing to Start Small

While pro-life teaching should happen from the pulpit, realistically it may have to begin with you. Never burden a pastor with additional work before you have demonstrated a willingness to initiate and share the load. The last thing a pastor wants to hear is, "Do you know what *you* should be doing?" Instead, *you* do what needs to be done. The pastor will eventually hear of it, which might start an essential conversation. Be willing to start small.

A friend of mine thought that teaching basic apologetics in his church might fill a need, so he put the materials together, presented them to the pastor, and offered to teach it himself. He did a great job. Word got around. Almost immediately, another class invited him to teach. Before long, he had a waiting list of classes wanting to bring him in.

C.S. Lewis said that the reward for doing a good job was usually more work. So, craft material or take curriculum already available, master the content, and energetically teach it. Then take questions. Every time you teach, you will improve, word will spread, and instead of searching for opportunities, you may find yourself fielding requests.

Take Down the Great Barrier

The greatest obstacle standing between many a woman and the cross of Jesus Christ is the body of her preborn child. This barrier exists for many men as well. The church must inoculate its people against pro-abortion messaging, certainly. But throughout the body of Christ there are millions of people who are wounded and feel damned by past abortions. The damage will not be overcome and the sense of damnation will never get erased if pastors don't preach about abortion and the road back through confession, repentance, grace, forgiveness, healing and restoration. No generic sermons or teaching on general forgiveness will make a scratch in that wall; but specific, effective, and compassionate messages focused on the audience of the abortion-scarred can tear it down.

Revival in the church may wait upon millions of individuals being freed from abortions in their past, both men and women. The messaging must be intentional and the ideas interwoven into overall Scripture teaching that demonstrates a commitment to a biblical, life-affirming worldview.

Again, many resources exist. Your PHC has individuals trained in post-abortion counseling. Groups such as Deeper Still and Reassemble offer retreats to help people work through an abortion in their past. Even if you don't believe that you are the right person to help others deal with such a devastating life event, you can facilitate bringing that message into small groups in your church.

Whether you teach a coherent worldview on life issues to Sunday School classes, youth groups, small groups, or college/career fellowships, eventually your pastor will take notice. Sometimes, what can't be accomplished by a direct appeal to the pulpit can succeed through a willingness to start small. Do that. But most importantly, start.

...To The Street

When Christians are properly prepared, life messaging will flow naturally into conversations and friendships outside of church. Connections between people, putting a human face on pro-life claims and ministry, can be one of the most powerful ways to overcome advertising and social media posting by abortion advocates.

Use the Media

Messaging by Planned Parenthood and their allies remains a formidable force. They have funding that most pregnancy centers can only dream about. The good news is that the media is now more accessible than ever. Digital media has never been cheaper, which is both a blessing and a curse. A blessing because high-quality content can be inexpensively produced by pro-life advocates. A curse because high-quality content can be inexpensively produced by our opponents. The rapid expansion of the capabilities and accessibility of AI has yet to be fully felt. The tools are everywhere, so it's going to come down to content and live performance.

Anyone who can write prompts can use AI to create images, videos, music; anything that can be transmitted digitally is in the AI wheelhouse. But the acronym GIGO (garbage in, garbage out) remains true. No doubt you have seen some terrible AI videos featuring people with twelve fingers, bodies that pass through solid objects, uncanny and unreal faces, and mouths that don't sync with the voice track. But we also have examples of creative excellence.

Spencer Pratt, a Republican nominee in the Los Angeles mayoral primary election in 2026, is a case in point (or at least his fans are). They engaged in relentless AI-driven video production. Not all of it was a hit, but when legions of people simultaneously create content, the odds are good that some of it will catch on. Consider Adam Scheidler's "Everything is Awful" which riffs on the song "Everything is Awesome" from *The Lego Movie*. The ad featured Lego-looking characters and effectively used humor and parody to drive Pratt's message home: Los Angeles is crumbling under the current mayor, so elect me.[230] Charles Curran's AI campaign video presented Pratt as Batman and his opponents as comic book villains.[231] Each video received millions of views and pundits argued that the landscape of political messaging has been altered forever.

Guerilla campaigns, like those produced by Pratt's supporters, can work. Even if they don't ultimately lead to election, they can capture substantial attention. To be competitive, pro-life innovators need to produce plenty of solid video while knowing that the flood of media is so great that it can become ephemeral. Today's content is constantly replaced by tomorrow's. Back when the only interruption to a narrative was a TV commercial, cultural analyst Neil Postman observed:

> There is no murder so brutal, no earthquake so devastating, no political blunder so costly that it cannot be erased from our minds by a newscaster saying, "Now, this." The newscaster means that you have thought long enough on the previous matter (approximately forty-five seconds), that you must not be morbidly preoccupied with it (let us say, for ninety seconds), and that you must now give your attention to another fragment of news or a commercial.[232]

The Internet and social media have created Postman's "Now, This" on steroids. Gaining traction is tough. Pro-life advocates can't ignore digital media, but they shouldn't rely on it exclusively, either.

Put a Face to an Organization

We commonly hear that people often have time or money, but not both. Money buys media, but time can purchase personal connection.

Yes, it's time-consuming to stand in front of one group after another and make your case for life. But putting a face to an organization, such as a pregnancy center, can go a long way toward helping women locate a PHC when they find themselves in an untimely pregnancy. Some might be convinced to contact an organization they heard about in an ad; but they would be far more inclined to call the friendly and informed woman who spoke to their group, providing contact information using a QR code that she encouraged everyone to save on their phone.

Direct contact groups, such as Created Equal or Protect Life Michigan, are excellent examples of street-level messaging. While both produce good media (you can find examples in Reels, on X, and YouTube) these videos are often simple clips of individuals interacting with students on college campuses and with others elsewhere. The media increases reach, but the people these advocates talk to "in real life" have a much deeper experience. They don't scroll to the next video or click on another link; there's an actual live person engaging with them. Maybe you see Mark Harrington standing in front of photographs of aborted children and asking, "So, what do you think about abortion?" The encounter reverberates far beyond the initial interview. It becomes the content for discussions at the university cafeteria, in dorm rooms, and likely in classrooms.

People sometimes change their minds on the spot, rejecting abortion and accepting pro-life arguments. In one video, Protect Life Michigan advocate Joy Price encounters a student at Grand Valley State University and engages her in conversation.[233] The student begins by identifying herself as an abortion supporter; but following a brief series of questions about human rights, she changes her mind. Most students have never read or listened to a comprehensive argument for the value of human life in the womb. But they have been exposed to abortion talking points. Joy isn't a celebrity spokesperson for a company, but a regular person wanting to have a chat about something important. It's disarming. It's effective.

One instance of pro-life messaging is likely insufficient to create lasting change. But as life advocates regularly show up on campus, and their interactions appear on student phones on social media feeds, these messages can take root.

Taking Back Former Life States

The quickest victories in moving a state hostile to the pro-life position to a life state are most likely to occur in states that, until recently, had life-affirming laws in place.

Pray for Missouri

Missouri is making the quickest attempt at a turnaround. The state fell to a constitutional amendment making abortion a right in 2024, but just two years later, a ballot initiative qualified to overturn that mistake.

At the time of this writing, the result is unclear, so if you are reading before November 2026, please pray for Missouri. If Missourians choose life, it will be a great victory. But even if they do not, the numbers are close enough to make subsequent efforts both necessary and worthwhile. So continue praying.

In every state, inoculating people against abortion advocacy must happen year-round, every year. Abortion advocates are both persistent and zealous. Only when we are as determined to save lives as the abortion industry is to snuff them out, will lasting change take place. It begins with a commitment to counter-messaging and consistent pushback, which lays the intellectual and emotional groundwork.

But that alone won't liberate former life states from legalized intentional child-killing. For that to happen, we need a coherent political strategy.

One Sample

Many predicted that Florida would join other states in making abortion a constitutional right—and it almost happened. Fifty-seven percent of voters approved Amendment 4. The only reason Florida did not fall was its high threshold for amending the constitution: sixty percent. Because it was so close, expect abortion advocates to try again soon.

Some of the strategies developed to secure Amendment 4's defeat were created by nimble, innovative pro-life advocacy groups. Working on a shoestring budget, Apologetics, Inc. recorded short videos. Michael Sherrard admitted in an interview: "We were bartering with Chick-fil-A coupons. I think we spent around $7,500 to make the videos and had no money for marketing, so we used our network of relationships to get the word out."[234] Partnering with the Colson Center, Summit Ministries, and their own church network, the videos spread. Florida Governor Ron DeSantis' office of Faith and Community came alongside to help with strategy and dissemination.

Using Apologetics, Inc.'s own speakers, as well as apologists from Life Training Institute, the video messages answered key questions, such as: "Does abortion actually empower women?" These videos also equipped viewers to make a persuasive, easy-to-use, 1-minute case for why Amendment 4 should be rejected. It also exposed the vague language of the amendment, demonstrated how young voters were being lied to, and explained why the involvement of pastors and churches was crucial. Tony Dungy, Super Bowl-winning football coach, was recruited to provide key arguments against the amendment.[235]

Some churches chose to play the videos for their congregations, pastors spoke up from the pulpit, and the message resonated enough to win. But it was close. Instead of waiting until the wolf is at the door, strategic long-range planning is essential.

A Bold Campaign

Fortunately, other innovative pro-life organizations with verified street credibility in messaging are developing full-fledged campaigns that you can help to deploy. Trevor Polo, executive director of Protect Life Michigan, created Operation Zero, a carefully-crafted strategic persuasion campaign and tested it out in Novi, Michigan.[236] The project ran from March to August 2024 with a goal of changing voters' attitudes and voting proclivities. Note that the voting-age population of Novi, MI is about 38,000 people. After Operation Zero's persuasion campaign, 5,200 voters reported abandoning the "strong pro-choice" voter category. Support for abortion decreased 4.7% and support for an abortion ban increased by 3.26 percent – representing a net swing of nearly eight percent toward banning abortion in the target area. And the program was just getting started.

Mark Harrington and his organization Created Equal was one of the first groups that reproduced Operation Zero. In 2025, they piloted Make Abortion History, a two-phase strategy designed to repeal Issue 1 in Ohio and safeguard children in the womb.[237]

Make Abortion History begins by identifying "persuadable" voters in key populations. In any voting group, you will find a smaller group of individuals who are ideologically committed to abortion, which no argument of any kind will sway. The good news is that a large plurality of voters—in some areas, forty percent or more—fall into the "mushy middle." These people are the key target. Moving just some of them can have a tremendous impact at the polls.

Persuadable voters become the focus of targeted videos and advertisements that address the abortion issue head-on. At this point, many political groups might consider their jobs complete. Make Abortion History, however, launches a second persuasive wave. It's not digital, but personal. The digital outreach begins to open persuadable voters to the idea that abortion isn't just "Wrong for Ohio," it's simply wrong. Then teams of advocates fan out in the targeted communities, knocking on doors and holding conversations with voters.

The results of the pilot effort are encouraging, with significant attitude and policy shifts among the target demographic. After comparing pre- and post-test groups, a perception shift occurred of over thirteen percent toward a pro-life view and a ten-percent policy shift toward pro-life protection laws. The most compelling aspect of the initial study was that six months later, not only did the areas surveyed maintain their new pro-life commitment, but in some variables, the pro-life position increased over time. Immediately following the campaign, for example, a 7.8 percent shift occurred toward the pro-life position that abortion is not health care. Harrington notes, "Six months later, this had risen to an overall +21.2% net shift."[238]

> It is almost unthinkable that a battle must be waged for the lives of unborn children. But since we know that battle is real, we must use all of our wits and resources to win. Under no circumstances can we accept failure.

One possible reason for the increase is that those persuadable voters who shifted allegiance engaged in low-level persuasion of their own. For example, many placed pro-life signs in their front lawns, signs that were still visible a full year after the pilot campaign concluded. Sometimes, merely "planting a flag," making a simple pro-life claim, is enough to get others to consider switching or to provide courage to weaker-willed voters to publicly stand up.

The campaign and the survey methodology continue to be refined in order to better identify "persuadable" voters and craft the right combination of messaging to increase already positive results. In reading the initial report, one variable stands out: the largest percentage shifts occurred among people in the pre-test who identified completely with the pro-abortion position, but who, after encountering the campaign and interacting with pro-life advocates, swung entirely to the other side.

Such results confirm the idea that most Americans have never been exposed to a comprehensive case for life. They caught their current position like a person catches the measles; they simply got it from someone else. But once exposed to the evidence and reasoning behind the pro-life position, when they see what abortion actually does to its tiny victims, many individuals become just as adamant about actively saving lives as they once were in favor of passively allowing them to be destroyed.

Winning the battle for the minds of voters in hostile states requires pro-life advocates to fight back with clarity, with strong, easy-to-understand, evidenced claims. After people know what is true, follow up with supportive testimonies of women who felt tempted to intentionally kill their own children but who rejected that path and chose life instead. Show the aftermath of what abortion does to the bodies of small children. Abortion advocates sell death, while pro-life advocates offer hope. Engage vigorously on the side of life.

Invading Abortion States to Change the Culture

In 1865 London, William and Catherine Booth began to minister to drunkards, thieves, and prostitutes. They wanted to lead them away from their self-destructive existence to flourishing lives in Christ. Before the start of what they called "The Christian Mission," they went out, located, and trained evangelists who joined them to fight for the souls of men and women.

Imagine what would have happened had the Booths thought, *Well, the people of London have finally turned their lives around. Our work is finished.* Had they done so, you likely never would have heard of The Salvation Army and its global impact.

If you are fortunate enough to live in a life-affirming state, thank God. The people of your state determined to pass life protection laws and value preborn children. But the last thing you should do is hide that message away and believe that because your own children are safer from abortion, your work is done. (They are not really safe in any state because of e-tail abortions and shield laws; but, God willing, life states will soon be free of interstate interference.) It's time to take the battle to the enemies of life.

Strengthen What is Weak

No state is likely to have every safeguard in place to protect all pre-born children. It will take time for some to pass appropriate human life protection acts, make changes in education, or alter the way boys and girls are taught in school. But once pro-life people sense that their state is trending clearly in the right direction, at least a portion of the support they offer should head across state lines to help those who live in underserved areas and abortion states.

Pregnancy help centers strategically located near the borders of abortion states are in a prime position to begin taking the land. Locate and coordinate with interested people across the border to plant new centers. Maternity homes, or host home projects, can be initiated. Every aspect of pro-life work that exists in relative ease in a state whose citizens already recognize its value can be reproduced in a death state. But it may need to be helped along.

I recall several trips into regions such as New England, California, or the Pacific Northwest, where center staff told me that that they worked in a "spiritually dark" place. They found it hard to develop support and impossible to engage many churches. Despite having the fierce faith that any ministry requires to succeed in hostile territory, some directors felt alone.

Think of what it would mean to a director of a strategically on-mission center, but one which struggles to get sufficient financial or material support because of its location, to receive regular, out-of-state funding from a center, a Sunday School class, or a group of concerned pro-life people who want them to succeed.

In addition to strengthening existing centers, we need more centers. Again, one of the greatest barriers to developing new centers in hostile territory is the difficulty involved in raising funds and staffing those centers. In the next chapter, I'll show you how to move ahead.

A Full-Time Calling

Despite the efforts of Scott Klusendorf of Life Training Institute, John Ensor of PassionLife, and me to find Christian colleges and universities willing to adopt even a certification program for individuals interested in pursuing pro-life advocacy and pregnancy help center work, to date we have held these programs on only two campuses.

With more than 2,700 pregnancy help organizations in the U.S. and many national, state, and local advocacy groups, I would hope that a Christian campus would jump at the chance to be the first to host a permanent certification or bachelor's program. We have the curriculum and will, initially, provide the instruction. If you know any high-level administrators at a Christian college or university whom you think might have interest in making this program happen, please have them contact me. In the meantime, Klusendorf and I are talking about creating an academy where such training could take place; call it a "trade school" for pro-life advocates and center professionals. Pray with us as we consider next steps.

"If you build it, they will come" works only in the movies. Making professional-level training happen will require a dedicated initial cohort. Many center directors come to their work at mid-career or later. If you are a young person completing high school or college, or if you know such a student, pray and seek counsel about committing your professional career to life-affirming work. If you want to see hostile territory won for life, especially if you are young and mobile, consider being willing to relocate to fight where the battle is hottest. Whether as an advocate or in PHC work, you will be a missionary on a fertile field in every sense of those words.

Even in the most spiritually dark areas of our nation, setting up a PHC or working with advocacy organizations brings light, especially when they work alongside churches. It may be true that some clients who become convinced during counseling that their preborn child's life is worth saving, may still reject Christ's offer of salvation (at least initially). But even they will recognize life as the superior value over a culture of death. Life over death is an idea that J.R.R. Tolkien might have recognized as *protoevangelium*, something that works as a precursor to (or a kind of "first telling" of) the gospel, tilling up the hard ground and preparing it for seeds.[239]

Sharing and spreading the truth about life, recounting stories of children saved—these kinds of experiences lay the foundation for behavior and policy change. It is arduous, emotionally-taxing work, so not for the faint of heart. Abortion states cannot be abandoned. The number of individuals speaking out for the lives of their preborn neighbors is few. But you can be a Hebrews 12:1 believer, part of the "great cloud of witnesses" (explored in Hebrews 11) that enables individuals to continue their difficult work despite the Enemy's efforts. You can be a Philippian, commended for supporting the work of the gospel in cities and nations not their own.[240] *Every* act of support, *every* voice, *every* set of hands that can do the work will save lives and bring glory to God.

The Final Pivot

When I train public speakers, I introduce them to Monroe's Motivated Sequence, an organizational structure designed to move people to take action. The steps are attention, need, satisfaction, visualization, and action.

First, you gain your audience's attention at the start of the introduction, then, in your first major point, you explore the problem they face (their need). Next, offer a solution or solutions to fix it (satisfaction). Many students want to stop there, thinking, "wait, I explained the problem and solved it, so I'm done!" Not so fast.

If I want to discuss the problem of encroaching wastewater seeping across the border of Mexico and into San Diego, I might argue that the solution would be to build a transnational sewage treatment plant. How many people in my audience do you suppose would have the technical acumen or the money to single-handedly build such a plant? Statistically, zero. Just knowing a solution exists does nothing to bring it about.

But individuals listening to that presentation can hear what life would be like if such a plant existed: cleaner, bluer water, and safer beaches for their children to play on (visualization). And they can be offered concrete steps they could take to help make the solution a reality (action). Perhaps they could donate to a fund, write letters lobbying representatives to spearhead building the plant, form an exploratory or fact-finding group to look at making the solution feasible, or create mitigation plans to help in the interim. Any and all of these actions represent moves toward fixing the problem.

Forward, March

I promised in the introduction that this book would not merely explore the nature of the difficulties pro-life advocates face in the *Dobbs* era. I devoted only the first few chapters to that analysis. Every other chapter has provided pivots: shifts we can take to move us closer to building states, and eventually a nation, that welcomes preborn children into the culture and protects them in the law.

In these last two chapters, I will explore final strategies and lay out concrete action steps that you and others can take to transform these solutions into reality.

PIVOT

5

FROM INTENTION TO ACTION

CHAPTER 13

The Difference It Makes When You Do Something

My father, Bud, was a decorated combat veteran, a Lt. Colonel in the United States Marine Corps, 6'7" and 250 pounds. He had authority. He had command. He knew how to get stuff done. And because he wanted his boys to learn how to navigate the problems of life, he educated us. Much of his instruction he delivered in the form of short, military proverbs (some of which I don't think I could share here). He called them "Newmanisms." Here are three important ones:

"If you can read, you can do anything."

"'Can't' never did anything."

"If something is worth (complaining) about, it's worth doing something about."

My father was trying to teach us that if we could know the truth, rightly assess our abilities, and engage our wills to act, we could overcome obstacles and achieve our objectives. That same spirit motivated the writing of this book.

You have read, so you know the truth about what you're up against. You've seen a lot of solutions, so you know that everyone can do something. And if, in reading about the ongoing battle for life, you recognized that intentional child-killing must stop, then you have an obligation to do something about it. Therefore, I want to help you pivot from good intentions toward action.

Intention and Action

Social media has turned far too many people into serial virtue signalers. Use the right overlay on your Facebook profile photo once news of a tragedy or injustice breaks, and you can instantly communicate your tribal membership, demonstrating that you are to be counted among the "good people." It doesn't actually require you to *do* anything for the victims or to provide material support for the cause. In most instances, the issues about which people signal on social media are so geographically distant ("standing with" the people in Ukraine or Gaza, for example) that it's virtually impossible for the signaler to do anything practical. But indicating intentions, telling everyone what you *would* do if you *could* (even though you know you *can't*) is enough to induce others to congratulate you. The dopamine hit of approval follows shortly thereafter. It may feel good, but as a strategy it fails. The New Testament story about two sons and a vineyard has something to say to us:

> But what do you think? A man had two sons, and he came to the first and said, "Son, go work today in the vineyard." And he answered, "I will not"; but afterward he regretted it and went. The man came to the second and said the same thing; and he answered, "I will, sir"; but he did not go. Which of the two did the will of his father? (Matthew 21:28-31)

The story turns not on intention, but action. The first son did not intend to go (and he told his father so), but then regretted it and did the work. The second son may have intended to go, or he may just have been virtue signaling to his dad by saying he would. The fact remains that he did not go. Regarding the will of their father and the work needing to be done, intention didn't matter. Action did.

Much of this book contains stories and examples that may have been tough to read. As you read, you likely felt astonished, angry, even disbelieving. The injustice of intentional child-killing (once you accept it as the appropriate definition for elective abortion) is glaring. But emotional responses alone rarely fuel consistent action. And the longer you wait to act, after feeling the urge to do something, the less likely you will ever take action.

Recognize the good intentions present within you now. As you read the following pages, make a commitment: "I will choose, at minimum, one of the actions represented here and engage my will to do it." What follows is not an exhaustive list of actions designed to advance the cause of life, but it will give you plenty of actions to choose from. Where you begin may not ultimately be where you end up. Starting, however, is the necessary first step. As preachers like to say, "God can't steer a parked car." Look over these recommendations, choose at least one, and get started.

All Individuals

Regardless of who you are or where you live, you can do *something*. You can pray. You can set an example. You can join others. Don't merely intend something good; do it.

Pray

When some individuals see prayer at the top of a to-do list, they immediately think, *That's the one for me!* They reason that it appears easy and costs little—but that is not *remotely* how I would like you to think about agreeing to pray. I have two reasons.

First, God takes prayer commitments very seriously. When you promise to pray for someone, you are telling them that you will go regularly before Almighty God on their behalf. When I make such a promise to an organization, I make sure to put a start and stop date on my commitment. Victoria Robinson, part of an organization named Reassemble that helps people to overcome the woundedness caused by abortion in their past, asked me to be a part of her prayer team. I agreed to do so for one session. When she asked me to "re-up," I politely declined—not because her mission isn't important, but because I knew I was in the middle of a big project of my own (this book) and I couldn't commit the time.

If you ever feel tempted to think that agreeing to pray for a pro-life organization will be easy, think again. *Carefully*. If you are a confirmed prayer warrior, you know what you're signing up for and I would encourage you to go ahead.

Second, when I ask members of my audience at a fundraising event to pray for the organization, I tell them that I don't want them to pray "if," but "how." I don't ask them to go before God to determine whether they should become involved in the work of the pregnancy help center. They've already heard what we are up against and why it matters, and such knowledge brings obligation. I want them to pray about how they can use their time, talents, and resources to stand in the gap alongside this center on behalf of the lives of preborn children at risk of being intentionally killed.

Prayer is neither easy nor without cost. It is an integral part of the spiritual battle being waged *right now*.

Do What You Can Where You Are

Whether you're single, have a spouse, have children, or are part of a local church, the next action you can take is to set an example. You are part of some larger group, and everyone in that group is either influencing or being influenced by others.

Most people in this nation have been taught by academia, the media, perhaps even their own state, to restrain themselves about sharing pro-life views. If you're a man, you are told that "if you don't have a uterus, you don't get an opinion." Refuse to be silenced. Both male and female children are victims of abortion, but because of their current location they cannot visibly or audibly stand up for themselves. They need a courageous advocate: you.

Small actions can make a difference. You don't think of yourself as a public speaker, but you don't mind interpersonally talking to people?

There are ways forward. Some people like to go out in public wearing hats and t-shirts and so become walking human billboards for life-affirming messaging. Seeing statements like the following invites conversation:

"I'm part of the pro-life generation."

"Embryology teaches human life begins at conception."

"All children deserve a right to life."

"Pregnant? Scared? We can help!" (with the contact info of a local PHC on it).

Not only can you indirectly spark conversations, you can intentionally speak truth.

Read and reread chapters five and six on language. Refuse to adopt the terms used by abortion advocates. Use the word "abortion" only if you define it first: "an act of violence that intentionally kills a child in the womb." Don't talk about fetuses and embryos unless you're in an embryology or biology class. In conversation, the human being in a woman's womb is always a "child."

It may take a while to adopt a new way of speaking, but be aware of the words you choose. You might role play with others until it becomes natural. Expect some pushback, but don't allow your opponents to police your speech. You have good reasons for adopting these terms, so always be ready to share them. Individuals using other terms should be asked to defend them. People who respond "It's a fetus!" should be challenged to explain what species that fetus is. It's a *human* fetus, the child of two human parents.

If you're a parent raising children, don't wait for a church or a school to teach them the truth about the beginning of life in the womb. Start at home. Read Scripture that talks about God overseeing the creation of children, knitting them together in their mothers' wombs. Talk through what it means that John the Baptist and the baby Jesus interacted with one another before either was yet born. Watch the baby Olivia video together and talk about it. Marvel together as you watch how a zebra fish's nervous system grows; there is a time-lapse video of that process (unfortunately, often mislabeled as a human embryo).[241] The latter isn't a video of a child in the womb, but the system development is similar and amazing. As children grow older, reinforce their understanding that human life begins at conception. Introduce them to the arguments advanced by abortion advocates; don't wait for pre-teens to encounter them for the first time from friends or social media. Evaluate those arguments using Scripture, science, and moral reasoning.

In other words, inoculate them against abortion advocacy so that when they inevitably encounter it, they will be prepared. As you educate your children, you receive the bonus of learning yourself.

Join to Speak Up and Rescue

Educating yourself and your family is foundational, but to protect the lives of preborn children requires coordinated effort that goes beyond the home. No need to reinvent the wheel here; much of the infrastructure required to defeat abortion advocates already is in place. But to succeed, it requires additional volunteers, staffers, and resources. Read what follows, choose, and then act.

Give Your Time

Many individuals recoil at the idea of "volunteering," seeing it as a kind of involuntary servitude where someone shows up to do random jobs. That's not how it works at most of the life-affirming organizations I've interacted with. Instead, they want to match the interests, skills, and experience of volunteers to the needs of the organization. One case in point: Board Members.

Every non-profit organization needs a board of directors, individuals who provide oversight and direction to the ministry. When PHC directors talk with me at an event about asking for board members, I advise them to ask for individuals with specific skills. Many people, who like the idea of being on a board, put themselves forward thinking that they will do some good and maybe get a hit on their resume. I tell directors, "You don't want board members; you want problems solved."

Ministries have diverse challenges that morph as they progress through various stages of development. PHCs in a building phase might benefit from having a commercial realtor or general contractor on the board. At other times, having an attorney, accountant, marketing specialist, or pastor might be necessary. If you're a professional, identify the skills you have to offer, then contact and see whether they might be a good fit for an area PHC or advocacy group. You might first want to offer to serve as a volunteer. That way, both you and the organization can see if you are a good fit.

Single Jobs

A pregnancy help center in Pennsylvania outgrowing its facility operated in a residential neighborhood inside a beautiful old house with an unattached garage. Moving to gain more space would be expensive, time-consuming, and would require an awareness campaign to inform the community about its new location. So, at the group's annual gala, we asked for tradespeople to step up—and did they ever. I recall getting a fun email that read, "The sound you hear in the background, the sawing and hammering, is from the contractor and workers who are building a connector between our center and the garage. It will hold two additional counseling rooms and a library." When people were made aware of the need, a skilled tradesperson decided to fill it. The project had clear start and stop dates.

Many opportunities to serve within pro-life organizations are one-off, single jobs. People donate design and printing services for a special event, replace rickety entrance stairways, refresh landscaping, assemble and deploy a painting crew, upgrade security, build custom bookcases, install or update software, and, in one instance, a guy brought in an excavator and placed two septic tanks for a new maternity home.

Every pro-life organization has a to-do list that it worries will never get done. If you have professional-level skills that you are willing to donate to complete a particular, well-defined task, then make contact and offer your services. Smart directors will get back to you quickly, fill you in on what needs to be done, or thank you for the offer and put you in their file for later consideration.

Ongoing Service

When a newsletter arrives carrying a breathless description of some titanic victory, nothing feels better than to know you were a part of it. While some organizations run entirely on paid staff, many still rely on people who show up to do work. The reward is watching the change in people's lives and in the culture.

Start Young

When my sons were quite small, they accompanied my wife, Sharon, to our area PHC once a month to help prepare newsletters for mailing. They would sit at a table, carefully seal them, and apply address labels (today, this job is likely performed by machine, an indication of how long ago this occurred). Both boys were a part of something bigger than themselves, were "paid" with goodies, and gained several wonderful grandmotherly figures to speak into their lives.

Trained professionals aren't required for every job. For some tasks, volunteer workers don't even need to be adults. Make service part of your family dynamic.

Liaisons

As noted above, virtually every pro-life organization and PHC needs closer connection with churches in its service area. You might think, given the life-saving and evangelistic work these groups accomplish, that a tight relationship would already exist. Sadly, that is rarely the case.

If you are embedded in your local church and are a friendly, gregarious person who likes to talk to people, is good at taking notes, and can condense information well, you could be an excellent church liaison. Every church needs one, so if no one at your church has ever made you aware of a pro-life organization in your area, chances are great that you could be that representative. Contact organizations you'd like to work with and see if you could fill that need.

Digital Skills

Engaging in effective, life-saving work requires a wide array of digital skills. Often, too many tasks of all kinds fall into the lap of a director, who may be strong in some areas but weak in others. The ability to delegate is a crucial attribute in a good leader.

Many leaders in pro-life ministries are (I need to say this delicately) older. In other words, they are not digital natives. Many need help navigating social media and digital outreach. If you are technically skilled—and I'm not talking about people who merely post a lot on Facebook—perhaps you could fill this role. Understanding how to build search engine optimization, mastering an algorithm to increase visibility, and, increasingly, leveraging AI to produce outstanding content on a budget, are all important skills that must be regularly employed because the digital environment is constantly in flux.

Direct Engagement

Enjoy talking to strangers? Sidewalk advocates, canvassers (people who knock on doors to talk to others as part of a survey or political campaign), and people willing to interact with students on campus all have a place in various ministries. Some groups, such as Protect Life Michigan, Created Equal, and Coalition for Life, bring in interns and help them learn how to work effectively in these environments.

Organizing

Maybe you like to bring order out of chaos. Do you like to organize baby clothes? Virtually every PHC has an area where items from booties, diapers, and wipes to maternity clothes, cribs, and car seats are made available to clients. Donations arrive weekly and need to be sorted, stored, and displayed.

If you have a flair for visual presentation, every director I know wishes that their Earn While You Learn shop looked more like a lovely boutique. They want their clients to feel even more valued as they locate necessities for their new baby.

Other organizing skills include managing and securing records, materials management, and logistics and scheduling. If you have these talents, there is a place for you.

Education

One semester, I had a student trying to come up with a topic for an informative speech. I asked, "What do you do for work?"

"I'm an automotive mechanic," he replied.

"Could you teach people how to change their oil in the allotted time for the speech?"

"Everybody knows how to do that!"

I turned to the class and asked, "How many of you have ever personally changed the oil in your car?" Two hands out of thirty went up.

You may be one of those individuals who undervalues the knowledge and skills you already possess and which others need. Many people don't know how to do things that you consider common knowledge.

Education is an ongoing need both for PHCs and advocacy groups. They need people who can master the curriculum, teach it in an engaging way, and answer questions. Offer what you know and then see. You may be able to coach childbirth for new mothers, work with clients on nutrition, teach them to make a budget, balance a checkbook, craft a resume, study to pass a GED, or develop interviewing skills.

Many men also need these skills. See if your area center has a Fatherhood program. Some new dads don't know how to change a tire (or engine oil), use basic tools, or how to do standard home repairs. There is a place in the education space for nearly everyone.

Guidance

Emma is a nineteen-year-old college student in torn black jeans and a light blue t-shirt from H&M. Most days she has on light makeup, but this afternoon she looks pale and her cheeks are damp with tears she unsuccessfully tried to wipe away. She bows her head and her auburn hair partially hides her face as she trudges toward the entrance to Planned Parenthood. Despite the raised voices of the abortion facility's "escorts," Emma hears a young woman's voice plead, "I want to help you keep your baby. We can help you." Emma stops, pivots, turns toward the sidewalk counselor and challenges her, "Oh yeah? How? How are you going to help me?"

Scenes such as this one, on the street outside of an abortion facility with a group of sidewalk counselors, or inside a pregnancy help center in a counseling room with a woman who just received her positive pregnancy test, play out every day. The people interceding for the child in the womb and the life of the mother are called counselors or advocates.

No school I know of teaches this skill, but you don't need a degree in social work to be effective. Groups such as Coalition for Life and PHC staff will directly train you. What you need is robust commitment, a teachable spirit, and a compassionate heart. If you have those character traits, you might be an excellent counselor or client advocate.

Medical

Despite the incessant claims of abortion advocates to the contrary, the fact is that many pregnancy centers and clinics are licensed medical facilities. Since not all of them have the resources to hire medical people, they rely (to varying degrees) on volunteers.

Registered Diagnostic Medical Sonographers are frequently needed at many centers. Sometimes the difference between fewer and more open hours at a center depend on the availability of an RDMS. Some PHCs will train RNs to become RDMSs. Contact your local center and see whether your availability could meet their need. You might be surprised what a difference one four-hour shift twice a month can make.

All medical clinics require physician oversight. Medical specialists are also needed to read sonograms and prescribe progesterone to counter the fatal effects of mifepristone. If you are a medical doctor reading this, please pray about offering your services to your area PHC.

From Volunteer to Vocation

Phoebe started working at her pregnancy center in the baby boutique. Her organizing skills led to being put in charge of the annual fundraising dinner. She met a lot of people there and discovered she had a knack for donor development. The next thing she knew, that became her full-time job.

I once spoke at a fundraising banquet for a pro-life organization in Texas. Shortly before the event, I was informed that the executive director had abruptly left (people are human; it happens). I asked if they wanted me to add "Executive Director" to the list of things I would ask attendees to consider and they said "yes." When I finished my presentation, I drove to the airport and headed to my next engagement.

About a year later, at a national conference, a man approached me and said, "You don't know me, but I know you!" (I don't generally recommend this as a conversation starter. It's pretty unnerving.) He told me that he had been at that banquet a year ago as a business executive. That night, he couldn't get the call for an executive director out of his head. He and his wife prayed about it, he quit his job, and became that center's CEO. Many paths lead to full-time pro-life work. Most of those I know in this field didn't choose it, it chose them. Better yet, they will tell you that God coordinated the circumstances that prepared them to take on these roles at just the right time.

Many of the volunteer positions described above are full- or part-time positions with larger organizations. You may never have entertained the thought of a career in pro-life ministry. Perhaps you received this book as a gift for attending a banquet where I spoke and you are reading it as a courtesy to the director. But now you know. You can't seem to shake the image of young women intentionally killing their children in their dorm rooms or bathrooms, or of a performance artist screaming "I'm killing the babies" as she pantomimes an abortion. You sense the injustice when abortion states violate your state's laws by sending chemical abortion drugs through the mail.

The abortion industry is staffed with people whose full-time job is the destruction of children in the womb. The major cultural institutions of our nation are directed by those who devalue life. We must be at least as committed to saving the lives of preborn children as our opponents are to killing them.

So, you look at your training, you evaluate your experience, and maybe, you test the waters, first as a volunteer. Or you decide that the time is right to "burn the boats" and jump into the fray. If you sense a tugging in the direction of volunteering or seeking a vocation in pro-life ministry, please don't ignore it. You may be experiencing a divine appointment. At the very least, take some time, contact some advocacy groups or pregnancy centers, and explore what options may be available.

Many of us think we're ill-equipped or lack the option to volunteer for pro-life organizations. Fewer still ever move into a full-time vocation in this field. But it may surprise you to read that everyone, and I do mean *everyone*, can work to save the lives of children at risk from abortion.

Portable Work

"Wait a minute!" I hear someone cry. "You just said that not everyone can volunteer and most won't choose pro-life work as a vocation. And then you say everyone can work. What do you mean?" I'm glad you asked.

You give money.

When I say this to some people, they get a little sad, because in their minds, I'm just asking them "to write a check." But that way of thinking demonstrates a lack of understanding about what money represents.

Money is just portable work. You may be the kind of person who generates substantial income working in your field. The value of one hour of your time could be transformed into multiple hours of ministry. If you are a CEO, business owner, entrepreneur, consultant, brain surgeon, or contract attorney, a single hour might fund ten or twenty ministry hours. If this is true about you, maybe the best use of your time would be to generate a few extra hours a month and dedicate that work to a PHC or pro-life advocacy organization.

Maybe you aren't the person in these examples. That's okay. Most readers likely aren't. But everyone can give *something* if they understand and are committed to the vision and mission of the pro-life organization they support.

I embraced this view after a fifteen-year-old girl, attending a fundraising banquet I keynoted for a pregnancy center, told me that she came expecting to give fifty dollars; but once she knew the truth about abortion and the mission of this PHC, she felt moved to give five hundred dollars.

I don't ask everyone reading this to give ten times the support they currently provide (although maybe you can, or even more). But I *am* asking you to commit to give something now, then something monthly, and pray about what more you could do.

The Final Step

After reading of tasks to complete and roles to fill, I can't imagine that you haven't already found something you can do to begin making significant change right where you're located. If not, perhaps the next and final chapter will introduce you to prospects for ministry and service that will impel you to act. This is a battle, and it cannot be won unless champions for life step out and take the land.

CHAPTER 14

Giving, Going, Protecting, and Governing

Perhaps you once viewed pregnancy help centers and clinics as "local women's ministries." Far too many share that misconception. As a result, some centers have limped along on a subsistence budget for too long, negatively impacting staff retention and harming mission-critical operations. The generally-accepted statistic is that the professional lifespan of a center director is approximately three and a half years. You cannot win a battle when your veterans are constantly getting replaced by novices.

But now, you know different. PHCs represent the beachhead on the battlefield in abortion states. Advocacy groups are working to make cultural headway in states where, before the overturning of *Roe*, it wasn't possible. Like every other forward position in a conflict, they need resources, staffing, and support.

While the services and support PHCs offer are free to their clients, they aren't free to the center. Additionally, PHCs need funding to attract, recruit, and retain talent. In any enterprise involving people, nothing hurts more than constantly churning personnel. PHCs and advocacy groups are staffed by professional employees who have families of their own to feed, who suffer medical issues, require occasional vacations, and who need to plan for retirement. You want to see these organizations staffed by strategic visionaries, people who know how to get the mission accomplished.

Pro-life organizations should be able to organize and deploy talented professionals who know how to craft a campaign, do an ultrasound exam, counsel, do street apologetics, organize a center's logistics, or have the experience to talk to a scared young woman and lead her toward a life-affirming decision. PHCs need staff with emotional stability and spiritual maturity, who won't throw in the towel even if they need time to pray and weep after a difficult counseling session. Maybe they know that they are the last person who, after an ultrasound consultation, will ever again encounter that baby alive. I count running an effective PHC that produces excellent results as one of the most complex and challenging positions in corporate America.

Effective marketing to abortion-minded, abortion-vulnerable women takes technical and messaging expertise. Fortunately, some marketing firms now specialize in reaching those clients. Physical and digital advertising are required to penetrate the narrative monopoly that exists in most abortion states.

Getting the right people in positions of leadership requires funding. Procuring the needed pregnancy tests, supplies, and support, depends upon money. Creating and distributing messaging can be expensive . . . but the cost of failure is incalculable.

It just makes sense to give.

Giving Meaning

Providing personal financial support to your area PHC or advocacy group ties you to its mission and makes every one of *its* victories *your* victories. But don't limit yourself!

While pro-life organizations need financial supporters, I challenge you to become a champion for the work. Some people could put down this book, hit a round of golf with their buddies, talk about this great life-saving local organization, and raise more money than some centers bring in at an annual banquet. Others are connected through life groups, small groups, or youth groups; you could be the hero who makes a way for a PHC staffer or apologist/advocate to speak to those people. When they pass around support envelopes, be the first to fill yours out and include cash or a check. Others will follow suit.

In his book *The Wall*, Kirk Walden explains that if only twenty percent of the families who claim to be pro-life donated as little as $8.33 a month (and most could do much more), this seemingly meager amount of support would comprise over a billion dollars in annual resource increase for PHCs across this country.[242] That's *billion*, with a B. If you have never been a giver, become one today. Feel free to put down this book, locate your local PHC, and give. Most have a donor form or QR code right on their website, so there's no need to delay.

Here is an over-and-above challenge to the giver. If you reside in an abortion state, give to your local PHC and generously support advocates who speak for the rights of children to live. If you live in a life state, give to your local PHC, thank God that you live in a life-affirming state, and then choose a PHC in an abortion state and commit an amount to them. Perhaps you give generously to your own local center. Then you could choose a "*Wall*-level" gift of $8.33 a month in another state to support a PHC or advocacy group. In the next section, you will see how you might help form a new center; but right now, go ahead and act. The next paragraph will still be waiting for you when you get back.

Taking the Land

Judy Rouse directs multiple locations of a PHC in the Midland-Odessa area of Texas. A few years ago, I spoke on behalf of her PHC and, as often happens, I spent time on her main campus. Judy felt excited and proud of her center, but especially of her "war room." There on the wall was a map with a pin in it identifying the location of the center where we were standing. Out from that pin were more pins with some yarn around them, creating a circle. Another circle formed even farther out.

These circles represented a battle plan, Judy explained. They had planted their flag at the current location, had plans to take the land inside the next circle in the coming five years, and the territory in the next circle five years after that.

Ever since I stood in that room, I imagined a map of Texas. I know incredible directors such as Jana Pinson at the Pregnancy Center of the Coastal Bend in Corpus Christi and Nanda Kirkpatrick at Care Net Pregnancy Center in Houston. I keep imagining these directors in distinct geographical locations with their own war rooms, battlefield maps, and expanding circles of influence, growing outward until their circles converge and Texas is fully covered.

Then I imagine Erin Rogers at Bakersfield Pregnancy Center taking over the Central Valley and expanding eastward, along with Tina Williams at Alpha PRC in Maine moving westward. In every city, in every state, concentric circles expand and overlap, until every service area is covered and all clients have access to the life-affirming care that only pregnancy help centers and clinics provide.

I am beginning to see the same kind of strategic overlap between some of the advocacy groups with whom I work. The following are just two concrete examples of how you can help to take the land in a meaningful way.

Expanding the Territory

Throughout this book you've read about the tremendous work of pregnancy help centers and clinics. Even though more than 2,700 now exist in the U.S., about fifty percent of U.S. counties lack a PHC to serve their vulnerable populations. Since 2018, Heartbeat International, in partnership with local groups, spearheaded the creation of thirty-eight new centers in the U.S. (and an additional center in Australia) through their Pregnancy Center Life Launch program. Here's how you can be involved and how it works.

Maybe you live in an underserved area in a hostile state and want to see a professionally-run PHC planted there. Or perhaps you live in a pro-life state and want to see the benefits your community receives from their PHC extended across the border or into underserved areas in your own state. If you have the ability, you can directly donate thirty-five thousand dollars to the Pregnancy Center Life Launch program fund. But if you don't possess those kinds of resources, other avenues exist to make more centers happen.

Your Sunday School class, small group, or a bunch of like-minded friends can get together, you share what you know about the program, tell them about your support (no need to share the level), and challenge them to corporately raise that money (or a portion of it) and send it to the Launch fund. Then watch as Heartbeat transforms your generosity into another life-saving location.

How does Heartbeat do it? The ministry takes that thirty-five thousand dollars and uses five thousand of it to deploy its Affiliate Services Team to start a new PHC in an underserved area. Local residents raise thirty thousand dollars to support their new center—yes, locals have "skin in the game"—and Heartbeat matches that support with a twenty-thousand-dollar cash gift and ten thousand dollars in support programs, such as New Director and Board Training and Next Level Content Management Solutions.

Heartbeat could help to open ten new centers around the country this year if the Pregnancy Center Life Launch Fund received just three hundred and fifty thousand dollars. Once established, these PHCs build their own support base—and the fund moves forward to expand into new territory, plant more centers, save more children, and impact more families.

GITV in Action

You learned in the previous chapter about the Operation Zero strategy, started by Protect Life Michigan and replicated and refined by Created Equal with their Make Abortion History campaign. You can play a role in advancing this program to GITV (Get In The Voter) and work to make the passage of pro-life referendums, legislation, and state constitutional amendments a reality.

For example, Make Abortion History requires trained canvassers to knock on the doors of persuadable voters and engage in conversations about the value of preborn children and the need for laws to protect them. They seek people to distribute lawn signs. But most importantly, campaigns of this kind require funding.

In Phase Two, Make Abortion History expanded to five regions in Ohio. Running the program requires an investment of eighty thousand dollars per region, which means completing a five-region sweep would take four hundred thousand dollars. Some people who catch this vision can underwrite the program for an entire region. For others, a donation of two hundred dollars would represent a significant sacrifice. Does reading about the initiative excite you? Imagine how it would feel to be a part of it. Just about any reader of this book could pledge twenty dollars or more per month.

Many ways exist for you to support these campaigns to end elective abortion, create a culture of life, and bring healing to a desperately damaged nation. You will discover in Appendix 2 several excellent organizations doing a wide array of work especially worthy of your prayer, time, and financial support. If you aren't already convinced to act, turn a few pages to the appendix, review the offerings, and get started.

A Plan for Pastors and Churches

Contenders, written especially for pastors and teachers in the church, provides very specific guidelines for message formation. I aimed *Pivot* primarily at laypeople, but if you are a pastor and have made it this far, you've already noted several solution steps you can take. However, knowledge alone isn't enough. Churches, like individuals, must take action.

The first step many churches need to take may require you to build consensus among your staff, elders, and deacons. Most have never been exposed to a comprehensive case for life, and many cultural pressures might cause them to shy away from addressing abortion head-on. For many staff people, the biggest barrier to overcome will be significance. There are many aspects of Scripture to teach, any number of spiritual formation principles critical for congregants, and endless programs to plan. Leadership must rightly assess the real, lasting threat that intentional child-killing presents to the congregation.

A target has been painted on the backs of your teens and young adults, and well-funded abortion advocates are coming for them. A significant number of older adults are secretly and silently struggling with abortions in their past that are stealing their joy, confining them in prisons of doubt, and separating them from Christian service. In some cases, past abortions stand in the way of someone coming to Jesus.

Begin with a staff-level Bible study on bloodguilt and idolatry (particularly Molech worship) and demonstrate the links to contemporary abortion practice. Then teach staffers to make the scientific, moral, and biblical case for life. Craft a plan to teach these Scripture passages and concepts and commit to weaving them into sermons and teachings every time the topic or the passage is adjacent to abortion: murder, life, children, idolatry, bloodguilt, mothers, fathers, sin, family, etc. Structured teaching builds an appropriate Christian worldview in your congregation that helps congregants withstand the persuasive propaganda of the abortion industry.

Commit to an age-appropriate educational program for your youth and young adults. Work together with parents to gain buy-in to the program. Help these educated believers understand the connection between their faith and what it means for the way they treat people experiencing untimely pregnancies. What they learn should influence how they vote and what they support. In other words, don't forget the action steps that will enable them to make a difference and reinforce the message they have received. Make sure the program is perennial, that it can be repeated and expanded from year to year. New people enter our churches monthly and may carry with them an unbiblical life ethic which, if unchecked, can spread.

Pastors will one day look back on the battle for the lives of preborn children with shame or gratitude. Shame if they saw the conflict and chose, instead, to abandon the field. Gratitude because they were granted an opportunity to save children and parents both physically and spiritually, and they grasped it with both hands.

Connect your church with your area pregnancy help center or clinic. Invite the director to speak to classes and study groups. Allow a representative to address the congregation from the pulpit. Put a face on the only organization in town that directly stands in the gap for the lives of preborn children. Investigate and then implement an Embrace Grace Program to build a bridge between clients who come to know Christ at the PHC and the discipleship of your church. Make sure your counseling staff and teachers know about the post-abortion counseling available at the PHC and of healing retreats offered through organizations such as Deeper Still and Reassemble.

If you prefer in-person training and educational help, I have an additional resource for you: Me. Over many years I have successfully taught more than a thousand pastors and thousands of laypeople through our Contend for Life conferences.

In the afternoon session for pastors and teachers, I explain why congregants reject truth claims from the pulpit, what pastors can do to strategically work around those obstacles, and why preaching and teaching about abortion differs from just about any other topic. Then I walk participants through message preparation.

In the evening, I teach a three-hour pro-life apologetics class, teaching laypeople and pastors how to make the scientific, moral, and biblical case for life; why abortion ideology places all human beings at risk, not only the preborn; and what they can do about it. You can find details at https://contendforlife.com. I would be honored to work alongside you to train your staff and inoculate your people against the abortion industry.

Dueling State Websites

Praying, volunteering, giving, and involving the church are all excellent ways for individuals and pastors to make significant changes. If, however, you happen to be connected to politics, governmental officials should do two things now: host pro-life websites and create strategic inter-state alliances. Both are largely symbolic, but symbols matter.

To say that California is committed to a comprehensive, aggressive model for government messaging from a pro-abortion state would be a gross understatement. The official California Abortion Access site (its logo makes it clear that it provides access "for all") lets visitors know that abortion is legal, protected, and private. A featured quotation from Gavin Newsom makes it apparent that California is a national, even global, destination for those who want to intentionally kill their children in the womb.[243] It contains specific links for those outside of California, immigrants and those in the U.S. illegally, and minors.

The California site helps visitors locate an abortionist, plan for and even pay for an abortion. For the Deaf, the American Sign Language video linked to the site makes the pitch for abortion using all of the standard claims: abortion is safe, common, and a medical treatment. But at no point is the target, the preborn child, ever mentioned. Even though it mentions trimesters, the term is never linked to the development of the child in the womb. (I can't help but ask: Why isn't this considered informational malpractice?)

The main page links to a sub-page outlining all the ways California champions abortion, including a link to a complaint form designed to target "fake clinics," the term it uses for what it calls "crisis pregnancy centers."[244] Ironically, the state licenses the very pro-life medical clinics it assails on its website. Angela Bennett, the CEO of the SCV Pregnancy Center in California, held a press conference in 2023 chiding the state for the "fake clinic" accusation. She then proudly held up her center's state certification as a licensed medical clinic.[245] Nevertheless, in the war of dueling websites, California wins, hands down, because its leaders know what they're about and are pursuing it ruthlessly.

The federal government, under President Trump, launched Moms.gov on Mother's Day, May 10, 2026. The site links directly to Option Line and its vast network of pregnancy help centers and clinics. The site has a clear intent; its top paragraph tells visitors that the site addresses "the needs of mothers and fathers who face difficult or unexpected pregnancies."[246] If a pro-life Republican president succeeds President Trump in 2028, the website likely will continue. If, however, a pro-abortion candidate wins, expect the site to be removed, or worse, replaced by a pro-abortion site.

Few pro-life states have created dedicated websites detailing their connection to life-affirming services. Oklahoma has one (www.oklahoma.gov/life), but all pro-life state legislatures should establish and fund a site. Before they start, they should have a good look at California's website and spend time developing sites specifically designed to thwart it.

Since most pro-life states lack a dedicated site, kudos to Oklahoma for making an effort. Still, the site has much room for improvement. Oklahoma's current landing page prominently features links to service categories for pregnancy, parenting, adoption, and financial assistance. The rest of the home page features a large video of the governor and his wife. The interactive map at the bottom leads visitors only to county health services. To find pregnancy help centers and clinics, you must click through on the Pregnancy tab. While a basic "Pregnancy Resource Center Locations" tab leads to a poorly designed PDF, the layout of the Pregnancy page does not clearly direct anxious mothers who might be seeking an abortion to the real counsel and aid they need to make life-affirming decisions. Visitors must scroll down and search before finding a link to the Oklahoma Pregnancy Care Network, where they will finally encounter a well-designed page complete with a Nurse Chat feature at the bottom.

Texas Family Resources, another state-level site, presupposes that all women who find themselves pregnant are seeking services and not abortions.[247] The site is easy to navigate, but in its "services offered" filter one finds no listing for "limited ultrasound," something that a woman seeking to confirm her pregnancy might want.

State health departments obviously want pages that link to their various services. But if life states truly want to improve their outreach to women considering abortion, they need dedicated pages designed with abortion-minded/abortion-vulnerable clients in mind. I encourage their legislators to contact Heartbeat International to connect with OptionLine, and also with HopeSync. Many good pro-life marketing groups with long experience in this space could aid states improve their web design.

Few Websites, No Alliances

In chapter three I described the Reproductive Freedom Alliance, started by California Governor Gavin Newsom. Twenty-three governors feel so proud of their membership in this coalition that they allow their names and photographs to be displayed on the Alliance website, alongside tabs linking to their achievements in supporting and expanding the intentional killing of children. Newsom leads with thirty-one tabs, with others not far behind.

Searching the Internet for "Governors abortion alliance" will bring up many websites and news stories about this infamous group of pro-abortion state executives. Some hits describe the group, others offer congratulatory pieces on individual governors once they join the Reproductive Freedom Alliance.

What happens if you change the search word "abortion" to "pro-life"? Here's the summarizer at the top of the results page:

> No multi-state "pro-life governors alliance" is described in the provided context; instead, it documents a governor-led Reproductive Freedom Alliance of 20–21 states (later including Arizona and Guam) formed in February 2023 to protect and expand abortion access after *Roe v. Wade* was overturned.[248]

Thirteen states have effective abortion bans in place. I call on the governors of Alabama, Arkansas, Idaho, Indiana, Kentucky, Louisiana, Mississippi, North Dakota, Oklahoma, South Dakota, Tennessee, Texas, and West Virginia to organize and fight back. Other state governors who identify as pro-life would likely be inclined to participate, even those from states where pro-abortion constitutional amendments have passed, such as in Missouri and Ohio.

It took one motivated governor, Gavin Newsom, to create the Reproductive Freedom Alliance. It remains to be seen whether one brave pro-life governor could start a life-affirming alliance of state governors; or, if that happened, if other state executives would join. I have no way to know with certainty how connected anyone reading this book might be to powerful state political figures. But if you are so connected, contact them, point them to Newsom's site, and ask aloud, "Where is our response?" Possible names for the new alliance might include Coalition of Life Affirming States (COLAS), Every Child Safe Alliance (ECSA), Life-Affirming Alliance (LAA). Governments have marketing teams; I'm sure they can find one that will test well with their supporters.

An alliance of pro-life governors could work together on legislative priorities. Strong state voices would provide a welcome antidote to the poisonous rhetoric from the mouthpieces of the abortion industry. Best of all, member governors would encourage their pro-life citizens and help them to know that their views are shared, and that many like-minded people will take a public stand on behalf of their preborn neighbors.

The End Is the Beginning

Even before the *Dobbs* decision came down—in fact, even before it was leaked—abortion advocates already were planning their counterattack. While the court's decision initially unhinged pro-abortion forces, they quickly moved to plotting. Meanwhile, pastors in some churches told their pro-life people to tamp down their enthusiasm, lest they be seen as uncharitable to those who saw it as their constitutional right to intentionally kill children.

Robin Marty provided a blueprint for the pro-abortion response in *Handbook for a Post-Roe America*. Planned Parenthood dropped its mask and told people to "be proud to be pro-abortion." Chemical abortions, fueled by e-tail and protected by shield laws, expanded abortion's reach in a way that few could have predicted.

And that's where you find yourself today. You live in a country divided between life and death states, in which abortionists feel free to lob abortion chemicals over the borders that divide them.

But there is a way out and forward.

You need to pivot.

Pivot from using the language of the abortion industry to concrete word choices that reflect the reality of intentional child-killing.

Pivot from assumptions that "all Christians" (or even "all conservatives") are pro-life, to intentional educational programs designed to inoculate people against abortion advocacy and advance a life-affirming worldview.

Pivot from complacency about living in mostly pro-life states to urgency, leading to the kinds of policies that not only craft good laws, but protect the state, its citizens, and its children from those who would harm them.

Pivot from indifference that takes comfort in the thought that "my state's children are protected" to an outward-facing battle plan that crosses into hostile, pro-abortion territory to plant pregnancy help centers and confront (door-to-door where necessary) and defeat the bleak idea that sacrificing children is the key to the good life.

Pivot from hand-wringing inaction to engaging your will, and to aid churches and politicians in their efforts to protect all children, regardless of whether they are in or out of the womb.

Wishing vs. Wanting

Everyone wishes; few people want. Wishing is easy. All it takes is a daydream. Wanting is hard. Those who want are required to see the truth, recognize a problem, create plans, strategies, and tactics, and demonstrate a willingness to sacrifice to obtain the goal.

I'm not asking, "What kind of world do you wish you had?" Instead, I'd like to know, "What kind of world do you say you want? And what are you willing to sacrifice to get it?"

You have the information you need, along with many of the tools required to start achieving that world *right now*. All that remains is for you to put this book down, or loan it to a friend and discuss it, determine what initial step you are going to take, and then do it. Delay is the enemy of action. The longer you refrain from doing what you must, the less likely you will ever do it. The wise person, once knowing the right thing to do, begins immediately. I am not saying that doing so will be easy. What God demands of you is faithfulness.

I can envision the world I want. It's a world that values the lives of all innocent human beings, from the moment of conception until a natural death. It is an achievable world. If it wasn't, I likely would have given up this battle decades ago. The truth of the message of life can win, even in what currently are the darkest, most savagely pro-abortion regions of our nation. It all begins with one person choosing to take that first action.

If you do, you will immediately become part of the greatest human rights movement in history, battling the most pernicious evil that has ever stalked the human race. Innumerable children, at risk of death but now alive, and countless parents – who will receive these gifts into their homes – will be grateful. And if delivering children from death to life is truly the endgame, who wouldn't want to be part of that?

Welcome to the battle.

APPENDIX ONE

What the Pro-Life Movement in the U.S. Can Learn from International Efforts

Pivot attacks the problem of intentional child-killing in the United States. The fierce battle has high stakes, but I believe victory is possible. While these pages lay out many strategies and tactics, it would be foolish to limit approaches only to those used in the U.S., especially when we have several groups with international experience. Because they don't speak solely within the context of western culture, their unique viewpoint helps pro-lifers in the U.S. to consider the conflict from a fresh perspective.

To that end, I reached out to two leaders in international pro-life ministries who could help reframe the issue. Both have been doing life-affirming work for more than forty years. They bring clarity of vision regarding abortion around the world. Their knowledge can help you see the battle for life from a global viewpoint that I hope will help encourage you as you find your own place.

John Ensor, the president of PassionLife Ministries, has a global ministry that reaches from China to Cuba (where his work was recently profiled in *World* magazine).[249] John is a pastor, pregnancy help center pioneer, speaker, and expert on pregnancy crisis intervention. He has authored many books, including *Innocent Blood: Challenging the Powers of Death with the Gospel of Life*; *Stand for Life* (co-authored with Scott Klusendorf); and *Answering the Call: Saving Innocent Lives One Woman at a Time.*

Raul Reyes is the president of Life Equip Global, which recently merged with Choose Life as its international arm. He served as the first Director of International Ministries for LIFE International and helped to found many pregnancy help centers and clinics. He has a passion for training pastors across the globe to develop a pro-life worldview and then multiply that message through effective preaching.

Marc Newman: What fact about international pro-life work would many Americans find surprising?

Raul Reyes: Many American Christians still think of abortion mainly through an American lens: *Roe*, *Dobbs*, state laws, elections, Supreme Court appointments, and local pregnancy centers. But abortion is a global crisis. I use the phrase "Global Abortion Genocide" because it forces people to see the scale of what is happening.

John Ensor: Less than 3 percent of all annual abortions worldwide occur in the USA. That means that 97 percent of the moral crisis of abortion is a world missions challenge. So, in 2010, I began teaching pro-life ethics, apologetics and pregnancy crisis intervention among networks of churches in China. Soon we expanded to other countries where abortion, infanticide and gendercide are concentrated.

Newman: Are there similarities between international and domestic pro-life work?

Ensor: When it comes to helping people in hard places envision how to rescue the innocent in their country, we showed pastors and lay leaders many examples, going all the way back to the midwives in Egypt, who rescued their baby boys from a legal genocide. Multiple examples through history get the imagination going, and the indigenous people soon begin to see what might work effectively in their culture and context. We also provided them stories and pictures and starting points from the pregnancy help clinics that have developed over the last fifty years in the U.S. They have learned much from the U.S. pro-life community.

Newman: But key distinctions exist?

Reyes: The U.S. movement has become highly professional, political, institutional, and center-based, while the international work is often more biblical, relational, pastoral, missionary, and multiplication-oriented. In the U.S. we are often responding to Planned Parenthood and the abortion movement, rather than simply seeking and responding to what God would have us do.

Ensor: Simplification is more life-saving than expertise. Education in western culture emphasizes expertise. Our books, our training manuals, our workshops all put value on providing more and more content and higher levels of understanding from experts so that we can be experts, too. But movements never grow through experts. Movements grow only when the message is simple enough to hear, follow and share with others rapidly. I took 800 pages of my books on Christian theology and ethics and reduced them to ten pages and four Questions. We trained one million Christians in China to stand for life in one month by teaching just enough and in a simple, clear way so that they could hear it one time, understand it, follow it and teach it to others immediately.

Newman: So simple is better, because it allows more people to be in the battle?

Ensor: The crisis is too great to think we can ever train enough experts. No, the goal is to teach millions of people just enough to know to act like the life-saving good Samaritan, and not like the Priest and Levite. We do need some experts. But like salt, a little goes a long way. What we really need is an army of teenagers, moms, pickleball grandmas, aunties, BFFs and everyday good neighbors trained up and ready to do four things: **treasure human life**, including life in the womb; **reject abortion** as the shedding of innocent blood; **experience God's forgiveness** of our past; and **rescue the innocent** one mother at a time, directly, practically and sacrificially.

Reyes: One of the most powerful things about international ministry is that it cannot depend on expensive buildings, large staffs, medical equipment, direct-mail fundraising, or Western-style non-profit infrastructure. It has to multiply through trained local leaders. The future is not simply "build more centers." It is "equip more churches." It is not only "hire more professionals." It is "train more pastors, women's ministry leaders, counselors, advocates, and volunteers." It is not only "serve more clients." It is "multiply life-giving ministries in every community."

Newman: A lot of pro-life work in the U.S. is centered on either political advocacy or the efforts of pregnancy help centers and clinics, but you both work with a lot of pastors.

Ensor: That's true. Anyone standing for life in any way is good. But rescuing innocents from being intentionally killed through abortion is permanent, even eternal. For twenty-two years, I sought to serve the Cause of Life in the US as a pastor, teacher, writer, and co-laborer with a focus on helping communities of churches answer the biblical call to "Rescue those who are being taken away to death; hold back those stumbling to the slaughter" (Proverbs 24:11). The most practical way for most of us to live that out was by developing and supporting a neighborhood pregnancy help clinic. Now that some of these pro-life services have developed in China, Vietnam, Cuba, Romania, Uganda and other places, based on lessons learned from the U.S., it is clear to me that they too have something to contribute back to the movement in the USA. For example, the pro-life movement, and especially the pregnancy help clinic movement in the USA is beset with leaders who are full of fear, make fear-based policies and are afraid of anything that might risk attack, criticism or potential lawsuit. Outside the U.S., Christians are trained in what we call the theology of the cross.

Reyes: Many pregnancy centers are doing wonderful work, but some are exhausted, underfunded, and overburdened because the broader Church has not been fully mobilized. The U.S. Church has had decades of pro-life awareness. What it needs now is pro-life responsibility. Not every church can run a medical pregnancy center. But every church can preach the sanctity of human life. Every church can train life advocates. Every church can identify women and families in crisis. Every church can support single mothers. Every church can disciple fathers. Every church can offer abortion recovery. Every church can teach biblical sexuality. Every church can support foster care and adoption. Every church can become a place where life is defended, welcomed, and restored.

Newman: So there is a need for pastoral and pro-life leaders who will risk and sacrifice.

Reyes: Some of the strongest pro-life leaders in the world do not have big platforms, major donor bases, political access, or national conferences. They are pastors, women, missionaries, doctors, counselors, and volunteers serving in places where the need is overwhelming and the resources are limited. That should humble the U.S. movement. We have much to give, but we also have much to learn. International leaders often understand spiritual warfare, prayer, sacrifice, family systems, community pressure, poverty, shame, and courage in ways that American leaders may overlook.

Ensor: In Russia, China, Cuba, Vietnam, and many other places I have gone, Christians have long ago learned that being attacked is part of Christian faith. They never even think about how standing for life might cause them trouble. Once they see that the preborn child is an innocent human being, and God calls them to rescue the innocent, they simple make peace with any suffering that comes with it. They have long known that true faith in God turns to courageous obedience under pressure. They have lived knowing that faithfulness to Christ is often enmity with the culture. They know, and we would do well to learn, that prolife work is cross-bearing for the child-bearing.

Reyes: If I were to summarize what the U.S. pro-life movement can learn from international ministries, I would say it this way: The future of the pro-life movement is not merely political victory, professional services, or institutional survival. The future is a fully awakened, biblically equipped, gospel-centered Church that rescues the preborn, restores the wounded, strengthens families, and multiplies life-giving ministry in every community.

APPENDIX TWO

Pro-Life Organizations: Find Your Place

There is a host of worthy pro-life organizations that are not on the list below. I determined to place on this list organizations whose leadership is directly known to me. So, absence from this list doesn't indicate anything more than I don't know the leaders personally. (I apologize in advance for any organizations whose leaders I do know, but forgot to include here.)

I am including links to the organizations and, for those reading the hard-copy version of this book, a handy QR code. Look through these organizations; click on the links of the ones that interest you. The purpose of this list isn't to satisfy reader curiosity, but to provide outlets for action. Pray not *if* you're going to be involved with one or more of them, but *how* you will be involved. The true measure of the effectiveness of *Pivot* is whether it has moved you to act. If you do take action, please go to https://contendforlife.com/pivot and tell me about what you've determined to do.

Pregnancy Help Organizations

Where do you live? I have no way of knowing, so you won't find your local pregnancy help center in this list, though I think that many are worthy of your prayers, time, and financial support. You can also offer to serve as a liaison between your own church and your area PHC. You can locate your area pregnancy help center by going to https://OptionLine.org and doing a search on your location.

Heartbeat International

Heartbeat International has started, or supported and strengthened, over 4,000 PHCs since its founding in 1971. They aid in the professional development of PHC executives and staff through an annual international conference. Would you like to see more pregnancy help centers get started? In chapter seven you read about Heartbeat International's Pregnancy Center Life Launch Fund. Find out more about the program and donate by going to https://www.heartbeatservices.org/life-launch.

Care Net

Founded in 1975, Care Net is a Pro Abundant Life ministry that empowers women and men considering abortion to choose life for their preborn children and find abundant life in Christ. They have more than 1,300 pregnancy centers in North America providing immediate support to their clients and helping them make life-affirming decisions. Support is also offered through mobile medical units, churches, and a national conference. Find out more, including how to support their work at: https://care-net.org/.

Preborn

Pregnancy Help Clinics offer limited ultrasound so that their clients can see live images of their children in the womb. At the end of her visit, the mother can take home with her what is, for many, the first picture of her child. Ultrasound machines are expensive, and that is where Preborn steps in. They provide ultrasound machines to PHCs that are in need of them. If you'd like to help make sure a worthy center has the capacity to offer ultrasound, go to https://preborn.com/.

National Institute of Family and Life Advocates (NIFLA)

Thomas Glessner is the founder and president of NIFLA, which serves over 1,800 pregnancy help centers and clinics across the country. Beyond legal counsel, NIFLA has actively defended PHCs all the way to the Supreme Court. Additionally, they offer education and training, including an annual national conference. They've been instrumental in helping countless PHCs make the transition from counseling centers to medical clinics. Find out more and see how you can help at: https://nifla.org/.

Embrace Grace

Amy Ford is the founder and president of this valuable organization that serves as a bridge between PHC clients and local churches. Their vision is for every woman with an unplanned pregnancy to have a church to turn to in her local area for practical, spiritual and emotional support. They are looking for 23,400 churches, strategically placed around the United States, to open their doors and hearts to women with unexpected pregnancies.

Here are ways to serve:

- Lead a Group - Lead a support group at your church for those impacted by unexpected pregnancies
- Become a Mentor - Become a mentor through your church for those impacted by unexpected pregnancies, or single moms and dads
- Be a Church Buddy - Be a friendly face at your church and help women, men, and families impacted by unexpected pregnancies feel welcomed, connected, and supported

Go to www.EmbraceGrace.com to find out more.

embracegrace.com/give

Abortion Recovery Ministries

A significant aspect of winning the state-by-state battle for life is dealing with the devastating impact of abortion grief. Millions of people are in need of forgiveness, healing, and restoration which comes only by confession and repentance. These groups educate and sponsor retreats where people wounded by abortion in their past not only find hope, but rediscover their voices.

Deeper Still

I've known Karen Ellison, the president of Deeper Still, for many decades. Her husband, Arthur, is a primary reason I am in pro-life work. Deeper Still is an established ministry throughout the U.S., they are also expanding into China, Taiwan, Finland, and other international locations. Visit their site at https://deeperstill.org. Once you are on the Deeper Still homepage, click on the Training link to discover how you could be a part of this vital ministry. If you need healing from an abortion in your past – they work with both men and women – click on Chapters or Find A Retreat. To support Deeper Still's mission to bring chapters and retreats to everywhere they are needed, go to: https://deeperstill.org/give/.

Reassemble

Reassemble is run by Victoria Robinson, a vital voice in the pro-life movement. She is the author of *They Lied to Us* and *They Lied to Us, Too* – books chronicling the stories of women and men who have been damaged by the abortion industry. Victoria provides healing retreats for women, men, and couples who have experienced or been impacted by past abortions. You can support Reassemble by going here: https://actintl.givingfuel.com/victoria-robinson.

Direct Engagement Groups

If you have interest in pro-life work that emphasizes one-on-one engagement, Protect Life Michigan, Created Equal, and Coalition for Life are organizations with proven track records.

Protect Life Michigan

Protect Life Michigan is reverse-engineering an end to abortion using persuasion strategies and young people. Their three core focuses are Campus Multiplication, Advocate Transformation, and Summer Deployments.

- Campus Multiplication reaches every college student in Michigan with the reality of abortion and changes at least 25,000 pro-choice minds on campus each year
- Advocate Transformation provides intensive trainings to mobilize thousands of young people to actively share the pro-life message with a million or more people each year
- Summer Deployments (known as "Operation Zero") allow Protect Life Michigan to make entire cities measurably more pro-life

Learn more and join the fight at www.protectlifemi.org.

Created Equal

You've read a lot about Created Equal in these pages and its mission to Make Abortion History. They train students to engage in conversations with college students and the public on the street. Created Equal is pioneering a strategy to change people's hearts and minds so that they can pass strong pro-life legislation and repeal pro-abortion constitutional amendments. You can join them in this work, or help by praying for and helping to financially support their needed work here: https://www.createdequal.org

Education and Advocacy Groups

Life Training Institute

Scott Klusendorf, the president of Life Training Institute, is a longtime friend and colleague. He is one of the most gifted pro-life apologists in the world, and this organization leverages his knowledge to bring a life-affirming worldview to students all over the country. LTI exists for one purpose: to empower others with the knowledge and conviction necessary to make a case for life that changes hearts and minds. If you want to see a pro-life ethic spread around the country, support this work by donation or by bringing their speakers to your area. https://prolifetraining.com

The Center for Bio-Ethical Reform

Gregg Cunningham, president of The Center for Bio-Ethical Reform, has been working to awaken people to the threat of abortion and euthanasia for decades. Projects include the Genocide Awareness Project held on campuses to engage students in discussion about abortion, euthanasia, and other human rights abuses. Find out more about what CBR is doing at https://abortionno.org. Use the QR code to see how you can take action:

Education Resource Fund

The Education Resource Fund is a treasure trove of images, videos, and resources to help people make the scientific case for life. Browse through the site and you will be amazed at the number and quality of materials you find there. https://erf.science/. Don't forget to hit the Donate button to help others access this needed resource.

Apologetics, Inc.

More than a pro-life site, Apologetics, Inc. is a clearing house for a number of topics about sharing the Christian message and worldview. So why is it included here in an appendix of pro-life groups? Michael Sherrard, president of Apologetics, Inc., was instrumental in getting high-quality speakers and video to help defeat the move to amend Florida's constitution to allow for unfettered abortion. The URL will take you to the site, but the QR code will take you to the videos. I'd ask you to not only support this ministry, but also if you live in a state facing legal challenges regarding abortion, work with this team to create messaging that works. https://apologetics.org.

Contend for Life

Contend for Life is one of my sites. There you will find the information you need to host a Contend for Life Conference. This one-day event consists of two sessions: "How to Teach the Toughest Topic" – an afternoon session to equip pastors and lay teachers to preach and teach effectively on abortion, and "Contenders: Making the Case for Life" – a three-hour evening apologetics session that teaches everyone how to make the scientific, moral, and biblical case for life, why abortion ideology puts everyone at risk, and what they can do about it. Find out more at: https://contendforlife.com.

International Organizations

The focus of *Pivot* is on the battle over abortion in the United States. In Appendix Two, however, I invited two friends of mine to discuss how their work with international pro-life organizations might help to inform the strategies and tactics in the U.S.. If you have a burden for children at risk from abortion all over the globe, here are two organizations worthy of your support.

PassionLife Ministries

John Ensor's global ministry reaches from China to Cuba – where his work was recently profiled in *World* magazine. John is a pastor, pregnancy help center pioneer, speaker, and expert on pregnancy crisis intervention. If you are interested in the global fight for life, consider working with and supporting PassionLife Ministries. https://www.passionlife.org/.

Life Equip Global/Choose Life Global

Leveraging technology to reach pastors and leaders around the world is the focus of Life Equip Global. In 2027, this ministry will merge with Choose Life and become Choose Life Global, but Raul Reyes will continue as the driving force behind this ministry. There are a lot of opportunities to serve here, so look through the website and determine what God may be calling you to do and your level of involvement. https://lifeequipglobal.org/.

Index

V

W

Z

Endnotes

1 If you recoil at my use of the term "pro-abort" or "pro-abortion," please note that I am using the terminology that the largest abortion institution in the U.S. now advocates for itself when it says, "Be proud to be pro-abortion.")

2 "Pro-abortion rights protest held in downtown Detroit over leaked SCOTUS draft," *WXYZ-TV Detroit*, May 3, 2022. https://www.youtube.com/watch?v=33uemaUU78A .

3 Eugene Declercq, Ruby Barnard-Mayers, Laurie C. Zephyrin, Kay Johnson, "The U.S. Maternal Health Divide: The Limited Maternal Health Services and Worse Outcomes of States Proposing New Abortion Restrictions," *The Commonwealth Fund*, December 14, 2022. https://www.commonwealthfund.org/publications/issue-briefs/2022/dec/us-maternal-health-divide-limited-services-worse-outcomes.

4 This terminology pre-dates *Dobbs* by a few years, but post-*Dobbs* see Catherine Rampell, "These GOP politicians aren't pro-life. They are pro-forced birth," *Washington Post*, May 10, 2022. https://www.washingtonpost.com/opinions/2022/05/10/republican-politicians-are-less-antiabortion-than-pro-forcing-birth/. And Nikesha Elise Williams, "Pro-birth is not the same as pro-life," *Jax Today*, May 9, 2022. https://jaxtoday.org/2022/05/09/opinion-pro-birth-is-not-the-same-as-pro-life/.

5 State of California, "California Abortion Access," 2025. https://www.cdph.ca.gov/programs/ohe/abortion/pages/home.aspx.

6 State of California, "California Abortion Access," 2025. https://www.cdph.ca.gov/Programs/OHE/abortion/Pages/getting-an-abortion/types-of-abortion.aspx.

7 Ibid.

8 Kendall@PlannedParenthood, "What are Crisis Pregnancy Centers?" *Planned Parenthood*, November 4, 2021. https://www.plannedparenthood.org/blog/what-are-crisis-pregnancy-centers.

9 Ibid.

10 "California Abortion Access," 2025.

11 Oregon Health Authority, "Information About Abortion," https://www.oregon.gov/oha/PH/HEALTHYPEOPLEFAMILIES/ABORTIONACCESS/Pages/info.aspx.

12 Oregon Health Authority, "Where to Get an Abortion," https://www.oregon.gov/oha/PH/HEALTHYPEOPLEFAMILIES/ABORTIONACCESS/Pages/abortion-access.aspx.

13 Reproductive Health Access Project, "How to Spot and Avoid Fake Abortion Clinics," May, 2023. https://www.reproductiveaccess.org/wp-content/uploads/2023/05/2023-05-How-to-Spot-Fake-Abortion-Clinics.pdf.

14 Washington State Department of Health, "Abortion," https://doh.wa.gov/you-and-your-family/sexual-and-reproductive-health/abortion.

15 Washington State Department of Health, "Plan for Your Abortion," https://doh.wa.gov/you-and-your-family/sexual-and-reproductive-health/abortion/plan-your-abortion.

16 Washington State Department of Health, "Avoid Anti-Abortion Facilities," https://doh.wa.gov/you-and-your-family/sexual-and-reproductive-health/abortion/avoid-anti-abortion-facilities.

17 See New York State, "Abortion in New York State: Know Your Rights," https://doh.wa.gov/you-and-your-family/sexual-and-reproductive-health/abortion/avoid-anti-abortion-facilities; The Office of Minnesota Attorney General Keith Ellison, "Know your rights to abortion and reproductive healthcare in Minnesota," this page is complete with an alarming "Consumer Alert" regarding PHCs, https://www.ag.state.mn.us/abortionrights/; Official Site of the State of New Jersey, "Find Reproductive Health Care Services in New Jersey," also includes a "Consumer Alert" regarding PHCs, https://www.ag.state.mn.us/abortionrights/; Maine provides a PDF, "Know Your Rights: Abortion in Maine," https://www.maine.gov/ag/docs/Abortion%20Rights%20in%20Maine.pdf; New Mexico's page "Abortion and Reproductive Health," contains a subsection titled "Steps to take when deciding if you want an abortion." All of the links in this section go straight to abortion advocates and providers, https://www.nmhealth.org/about/phd/phdo/arh/.

18 "Attacks on Churches, Pro-Life Organizations, Property, and People Since the *Dobbs* Leak on May 2, 2022 (as of 5/19/23)," *Family Research Council*, https://downloads.frc.org/EF/EF22F17.pdf.

19 FBI, "Most Wanted," June 10, 2022. https://www.fbi.gov/wanted/seeking-info/pregnancy-resource-center-arson.

20 DCNF, "Pro-Life Pregnancy Centers Still Awaiting Justice 3 Years After Firebombing, Vandalism Spree," *Maine Wire*, June 9, 2025. https://www.themainewire.com/2025/06/daily-caller-exclusive-pro-life-pregnancy-centers-still-awaiting-justice-3-years-after-firebombing-vandalism-spree/

21 "Pro-life pregnancy center vandalized with death threats," *Fox 2 Detroit*, September 23, 2022. https://www.youtube.com/watch?v=2CPZ3uD_lYo.

22 Emma Arns, "Kent State pro-life memorial vandalized, defaced with pro-Palestine messages, students say," *Campus Reform*, April 12, 2024. https://www.campusreform.org/article/kent-state-pro-life-memorial-vandalized-defaced-pro-palestine-messages-students-say/25173

23 Heather Vasquez, email message to the author, July 25, 2025.

24 Romans 1:28.

25 "MSNBC guest wants to make 'sweet love' to SCOTUS leaker," *Fox News*, May 9, 2022. https://www.foxnews.com/video/6305839099112.

26 "'An eyeball just fell into my lap' and other horrifying quotes from leaked abortion conference footage," *Texas Right to Life*, October 20, 2015. https://texasrighttolife.com/an-eyeball-just-fell-into-my-lap-and-other-horrifying-quotes-from-leaked-abortion-conference-footage/. These videos were available on YouTube but were forced to be taken down by a judicial ruling that found that the Center for Medical Progress violated recording laws. This is the same kind of undercover journalism that 60 Minutes has engaged in for decades, but when the abortion industry is the target, the rules seem to change. For fuller coverage of the horrific admissions of those in the abortion industry when they think they are speaking only to themselves, see Alexandra DeSanctis, "I Might Pull Off…a Leg or Two," *National Review*, May 25, 2017. https://www.nationalreview.com/2017/05/undercover-video-center-medical-progress-exposes-gruesome-abortion-practices/.

27 Ellie Muir, "Who is Crackhead Barney? Viral 'ambush interviewer' behind the Alec Baldwin phone-slapping incident," *The Independent*, April 25, 2024. https://www.the-independent.com/arts-entertainment/tv/news/crackhead-barney-piers-morgan-alec-baldwin-video-who-b2534597.html.

28 Kitty Alvarado, "*Dobbs* ruling gets mixed reaction from San Diego religious community," *KPBS 65*, June 24, 2022. https://www.kpbs.org/news/local/2022/06/24/dobbs-ruling-gets-mixed-reaction-from-san-diego-religious-community.

29 See also, Jack Howell, "Considering Our Place in Our Culture: A Pastor's Thoughts On *Dobbs*," *Trinity Blog*, July 1, 2022. https://trinitynorfolk.com/content.cfm?id=3317&blog_id=52. A collection of such comments may be found here: Mark Wingfield, "Here's what pastors said this Sunday in churches not celebrating the Supreme Court's abortion decision," *Baptist News Global*, June 26, 2022. https://baptistnews.com/article/heres-what-pastors-said-this-sunday-in-churches-not-celebrating-the-supreme-courts-abortion-decision/

30 Jasmine Mithani, Shefali Luthra, and Abby Johnston, "What Abortion Looks Like in Every State Right Now,"

The 19th, May 25, 2022, updated October 7, 2024. https://19thnews.org/2022/05/abortion-rights-restrictions-laws-in-your-state/.

31 "Chelsea's Fund helps people across Wyoming access abortion care," *Chelsea's Fund*, https://chelseasfund.org/.

32 "Building Power toward a common goal: abortion access for all," *National Network of Abortion Funds*, https://abortionfunds.org/.

33 "Care Not Control: Repression & Youth Resistance," *National Network of Abortion Funds*, June 10, 2026. https://abortionfunds.org/care-not-control-repression-youth-resistance/.

34 Michael Wildes, "Hundreds of Pilots Sign Up to Provide Transport for Women's Medical Care," *Flying*, July 14, 2022. https://www.flyingmag.com/hundreds-of-pilots-sign-up-to-provide-transport-for-womens-medical-care/.

35 Tessa Stuart, "Pilots are airlifting patients out of red states to get abortions," *Rolling Stone*, June 29, 2022. https://www.rollingstone.com/politics/politics-features/elevated-access-volunteer-pilots-abortion-1375732/.

36 Robin Marty, *New Handbook for A Post-Roe America*, (New York: Seven Stories Press, 2021) xviii-xix.

37 Mary Calderone, "Illegal Abortion as a Public Health Problem," *American Journal of Public Health*, 50.7 (July 1960): 949. https://www.ncbi.nlm.nih.gov/pmc/articles/PMC1373382/pdf/amjphnation00308-0022.pdf.

38 Marty. *New Handbook*, 74.

39 These examples are not arbitrarily chosen. They are examples used for infanticide by Giubilini and Minerva drawing from the arguments for abortion on demand. Alberto Giubilini and Francesca Minerva, "After-Birth Abortion: Why Should the Baby Live?" *Journal of Medical Ethics*, 39 (2013): 261-263.

40 C.S. Lewis, *The Great Divorce*, (New York: Macmillan Publishing Co., 1946) 121.

41 Matthew McDonald, "Abortion Makes Men 'More Free,' Pete Buttigieg Says," *National Catholic Register*, July 31, 2024. https://www.ncregister.com/news/abortion-makes-men-more-free-pete-buttigieg-says. It wasn't a one-off comment. Here he is in a video saying much the same at :18 into the clip: https://www.youtube.com/watch?v=zdjorJo5AvE.

42 Laura Coverson, "'Miraculous Birth' at Cedars Sinai Delivers Family Holiday Joy," *Cedars Sinai*, December 10, 2025. https://www.cedars-sinai.org/newsroom/miraculous-birth-at-cedars-sinai-delivers-family-holiday-joy/

43 Gloria Oladipo, "California woman delivers healthy baby after 'essentially unheard of' ectopic pregnancy," *The Guardian*, December 27, 2025. https://www.theguardian.com/us-news/2025/dec/27/california-woman-ectopic-pregnancy.

44 John Bowden, "Abortion hearing witness confronts senators Cruz and Cornyn over her near-death 'on their watch,'" *The Independent*, April 26, 2023. https://www.the-independent.com/news/world/americas/us-politics/cruz-cornyn-abortion-hearing-b2327684.html

45 Now This Impact, "Senate Judiciary Committee Holds Hearing on Abortion Access in the U.S.," April 26, 2023, 2:25:50. https://www.youtube.com/watch?v=7TDw6o0QSmM. Dr. Skop's comments come at 52:02.

46 Ibid. Dr. Skop's comments come at 2:01:00.

47 Meredith Heagney, "Justice Ruth Bader Ginsburg Offers Critique of *Roe v. Wade* During Law School Visit," The University of Chicago: The Law School, May 15, 2013. https://www.law.uchicago.edu/news/justice-ruth-bader-ginsburg-offers-critique-roe-v-wade-during-law-school-visit

48 Caitlen Gertz, et. al, ""Impact of Clinic Closures on Women Obtaining Abortion Services After Implementation of a Restrictive Law in Texas," *American Journal of Public Health*, May 2015. https://ajph.aphapublications.org/doi/abs/10.2105/AJPH.2016.303134.

49 Lisa M. Koonin, et. al., "Trends in the Use of Telehealth During the Emergence of the COVID-19 Pandemic — United States, January–March 2020," *CDC Morbidity and Mortality Weekly Report*, October 30, 2020. https://www.cdc.gov/mmwr/volumes/69/wr/mm6943a3.htm.

50 *UCLA Law*, "Shield Laws for Reproductive and Gender-Affirming Health Care: A State Law Guide", Last update December 2025. https://law.ucla.edu/academics/centers/center-reproductive-health-law-and-policy/shield-laws-reproductive-and-gender-affirming-health-care-state-law-guide.

51 Julianne McShane, "Telehealth Abortions Continue to Rise—Even in Banned States, A New Study Shows," *Mother Jones*, February 24, 2024. https://www.motherjones.com/politics/2024/02/telehealth-abortions-continue-to-rise-even-in-banned-states-a-new-study-shows/.

52 Marlow Lacen, "Teen's medical abortion puts Louisiana, New York leaders at odds as Landry signs doctor's extradition order," *KTAL Now*, February 13, 2025. https://www.ktalnews.com/news/louisiana/teens-medical-abortion-puts-louisiana-new-york-leaders-at-odds-as-landry-signs-doctors-extradition-order/.

53 Sara Cline and Geoff Mulvihill, "Arrest warrant issued for New York doctor indicted in Louisiana for prescribing abortion pill," *Associated Press*, January 31, 2025. https://apnews.com/article/abortion-indictment-louisiana-new-york-doctor-63ff4d9da8a9b592a7ca4ec7ba538cd3.

54 Sara Chernikoff, "As Supreme Court weighs abortion drug, a look at pill usage since *Roe v. Wade*" *USA Today*, March 28, 2024. https://www.usatoday.com/story/news/health/2024/03/28/abortion-pill-use-is-on-the-rise-graphics/73122605007/

55 Lisa Baumann, "Washington stocks up on abortion pills ahead of court ruling," *AP News*, April 4, 2023. https://apnews.com/article/washington-abortion-pills-stockpile-1c1c7c107882f7a25a181af79a1f6790

56 Heidi Moseson et al, "How Effective Is Misoprostol Alone for Medication Abortion?"

New England Journal of Medicine vol 3, 6(May 28, 2024). https://evidence.nejm.org/doi/full/10.1056/EVIDccon2300129.

57 Original label provided to the author by a private patient for a Misoprostol prescription 200 MCG tablet.

58 Paul L.C. DeBeasi, "Mifepristone Antagonization with Progesterone to Avert Medication Abortion: A Scoping Review," *The Linacre quarterly* vol. 90, 4(2023): 395-407. https://journals.sagepub.com/doi/full/10.1177/00243639231176592.

59 P.C. Ho et al., "Misoprostol for the termination of pregnancy with a live fetus at 13 to 26 weeks," *International Journal of Gynecology & Obstetrics*, December 2007. https://www.sciencedirect.com/science/article/abs/pii/S0020729207005103. This study notes "that fetuses aborted after 20 weeks may show signs of life after abortion."

60 Louise Adsett, "Babies are sometimes born alive after an abortion. Should they be saved?" *Mercator*, August 29, 2024. https://www.mercatornet.com/babies_are_sometimes_born_alive_after_an_abortion_should_they_be_saved.

61 See the current FDA label citing a less than .5% on the bottom of page 7: https://www.accessdata.fda.gov/drugsatfda_docs/label/2016/020687s020lbl.pdf. See also Elizabeth G. Raymond et al. "First-trimester medical abortion with mifepristone 200 mg and misoprostol: a systematic review." *Contraception* vol. 87,1 (2013): 26-37. https://pubmed.ncbi.nlm.nih.gov/22898359/.

62 Caroline Kitchener, "Alone in a bathroom: The Fear and uncertainty of a post-*Roe* medication abortion," *Washington Post*, April 11, 2024. https://www.washingtonpost.com/politics/interactive/2024/abortion-pill-experience-stories/?utm_source=rss&utm_medium=referral&utm_campaign=wp_homepage. The *Washington Post* link is behind a paywall. Alternately, free access is available (at the time of publication) from the *Anchorage Daily News* here: https://www.adn.com/nation-world/2024/04/11/alone-in-a-bathroom-the-fear-and-uncertainty-of-a-post-roe-medication-abortion/.

63 John Funk, "Nebraska woman charged with helping teenage daughter have abortion," *PBS News*, August 9, 2022. https://www.pbs.org/newshour/health/nebraska-woman-charged-with-helping-daughter-have-abortion.

64 Nathalie Kapp et al, "Medical abortion at 13 or more weeks gestation provided through telemedicine: A retrospective review of services," Contraception: X vol. 3 (2021). https://www.sciencedirect.com/science/article/pii/S2590151621000046?ref=pdf_download&fr=RR-2&rr=9d3898005fdf6a79.

65 Sruthi Chandrasekaran et al, "Outpatient medical management of later second trimester abortion (18–23.6 weeks) with procedural evacuation backup: A large case series," Contraception: X Vol. 6 (2024). https://www.sciencedirect.com/science/article/pii/S2590151624000017.

66 Ashley May, "Mom pleads with doctor to resuscitate baby delivered at 21 weeks. 'Miracle' daughter is now a healthy toddler," *USA Today*, November 14, 2017. https://www.usatoday.com/story/news/nation-now/2017/11/14/mom-delivers-earliest-premature-baby-ever-and-chooses-resuscitate-miracle-aughter-now-healthy-toddle/861386001/.

67 Dang Thi Ngoan, "Development of infants born prematurely at 26 weeks," *Vinmec Medical System*, February 26, 2026. https://www.vinmec.com/eng/blog/the-development-of-premature-babies-at-26-weeks-en

68 Ibid, Ho, "Misoprostol for the termination of pregnancy," 2007.

69 Blake Zwerling et al, "Society of Family Planning Clinical Recommendation: Medication abortion between 14 0/7 and 27 6/7 weeks of gestation," American Journal of Obstetrics and Gynecology, vol. 233, 4 (October 2025): 229 – 249. https://www.ajog.org/article/S0002-9378(23)00726-3/fulltext.

70 Kitchener, "Alone in a Bathroom" 2024.

71 Lois Lowry, *The Giver* (Boston, Massachusetts: Houghton Mifflin, 1993), 186-189.

72 "The Porn Phenomenon," *Barna*, February 5, 2016, https://www.barna.com/the-porn-phenomenon/.

73 Sara Wilson, "Abortion reversal ban survives test of Colorado regulatory board rules," Colorado Newsline, September 25, 2023. https://coloradonewsline.com/2023/09/25/abortion-reversal-ban-survives-test-colorado/.

74 Olga Rodriguez, "California sues anti-abortion organizations for unproven treatment to reverse medication abortions," *AP*, September 21, 2023. https://apnews.com/article/california-lawsuit-anti-abortion-organizations-5930c914385a49d6677905a6422ecbcc.

75 Carter Sherman, "New York attorney general sues facilities promoting 'abortion pill reversal'," *The Guardian*, May 6, 2024. https://www.theguardian.com/us-news/article/2024/may/06/new-york-attorney-general-anti-abortion-pill-lawsuit-letitia-james.

76 CALIFORNIA FUTURE OF ABORTION COUNCIL 2022-2025 Summary of Successes, n.d., https://www.cafabcouncil.org/_files/ugd/ddc900_1cd4b2b71fe44a1e8bdb3992e4301ba2.pdf.

77 Adam Beam, "California governor buys billboards in Texas, 6 other states to promote abortion services," September 16, 2022. https://www.ksat.com/news/politics/2022/09/16/california-governor-buys-billboards-in-texas-6-other-states-to-promote-abortion-services/

78 Amanda Ruiz, "California Gov. Newsom's campaign puts up pro-abortion billboard in Austin," *Fox 7 Austin*, October 10, 2022. https://www.fox7austin.com/news/california-gov-gavin-newsom-abortion-billboard-austin-texas.

79 Katherine Schwab, "Planned Parenthood designed a chatbot that answers questions about sex," Fast Company, January 24, 2019. https://www.fastcompany.com/90296325/planned-parenthood-now-has-a-chatbot-that-answers-questions-about-sex.

80 Repro Legal Helpline, "Abortion Laws by State: Tennessee," 2026, https://reprolegalhelpline.org/abortion-laws-by-state/tennessee/,

81 *Ineedana.com*, "Need an Abortion?" n.d., https://www.ineedana.com/,

82 Ibid. https://www.ineedana.com/estimate-abortion-costs.

83 Lily Böhlke, "Despite Telehealth Restrictions, Aid Access Gets Abortion Pills to FL Patients," March 8, 2022, *Ms. Magazine – Public News Service Collaboration*, https://www.publicnewsservice.org/2022-03-08/reproductive-health/despite-telehealth-restrictions-aid-access-gets-abortion-pills-to-fl-patients/a78128-1.

84 Lori Kersey, "Abortion pill campaign targets rural West Virginia, Kentucky gas stations," *West Virginia Watch*, August 18, 2025. https://westvirginiawatch.com/2025/08/18/abortion-pill-campaign-targets-rural-west-virginia-kentucky-gas-stations/.

85 Carrie N. Baker, "Billboards, Trucks, Gas Pumps, Newspapers and Even a Boat: Mayday Health Advertises How to Access Abortion Pills Across the South and Midwest," *Ms.*, August 22, 2025. https://msmagazine.com/2025/08/22/abortion-pills-mayday-health-billboards-south-midwest/..

86 Margery A. Beck, "Nebraska mother sentenced to 2 years in prison for giving abortion pills to pregnant daughter," AP, September 22, 2023. https://apnews.com/article/abortion-charges-nebraska-sentence-36b3dcaadd6b705ca2315bc95b99bdc1.

87 Gary M. Atkinson, "The Morality of Abortion," *International Philosophical Quarterly*, 14.2 (September 1974): 362.

88 Christine Rendon, "Hilaria Baldwin shares latest sonogram of her daughter as she awaits arrival of baby number seven with husband Alec Baldwin: 'There she is!'" Daily Mail, July 12, 2022. https://www.dailymail.co.uk/tvshowbiz/article-11006313/Hilaria-Baldwin-shares-latest-sonogram-daughter-awaits-arrival-baby-number-seven.html.

89 Nicolas Rice and Angela Andaloro, "Kate Mara Reveals She Is Pregnant, Expecting Another Baby with Husband Jamie Bell" *People*, July 10, 2022. https://people.com/parents/kate-mara-pregnant-expecting-second-baby-with-jamie-bell/.

90 Rom. 1:25.

91 Jordan Boyd, "Study: Rate Of Serious Or Life-Threatening Complications After Abortion Pill Is 22 Times Higher Than FDA Claims," *The Federalist*, April 28, 2025. https://thefederalist.com/2025/04/28/study-rate-of-serious-or-life-threatening-complications-after-abortion-pill-is-22-times-higher-than-fda-claims/.

92 Patricia Santiago-Munoz, "The truth about ectopic pregnancy care," *UT Southwestern Medical Center Medblog*, October 22, 2019. https://utswmed.org/medblog/truth-about-ectopic-pregnancy-care/

93 Paul L.C. DeBeasi, "Mifepristone Antagonization with Progesterone to Avert Medication Abortion: A Scoping Review," *The Linacre quarterly* vol. 90, 4(2023): 395-407. https://journals.sagepub.com/doi/full/10.1177/00243639231176592.

94 Ibid.

95 Joseph V Turner et al. "Progesterone after mifepristone: A pilot prospective single arm clinical trial for women who have changed their mind after commencing medical abortion." *The journal of obstetrics and gynaecology research* vol. 50,2 (2024): 182-189. https://obgyn.onlinelibrary.wiley.com/doi/10.1111/jog.15826..

96 Ibid.

97 Michael Gryboski, "Colo. pays over $6M to settle legal challenge to abortion pill reversal ban," *The Christian Post*, January 7, 2026. https://www.christianpost.com/news/colorado-to-pay-6m-to-settle-abortion-pill-reversal-ban-lawsuit.html.

98 Mary Anne Pazanowski, "Abortion 'Reversal' Speech Protected From NY State Regulation," Bloomberg Law, December 1, 2025. https://news.bloomberglaw.com/health-law-and-business/abortion-reversal-speech-protected-from-ny-state-regulation.

99 Quinn Welsh, "Abortion pill reversal providers challenge California over commercial speech at Ninth Circuit," *Courthouse News Service*, October 9, 2025. https://www.courthousenews.com/abortion-pill-reversal-providers-challenge-california-over-commercial-speech-at-ninth-circuit/.

100 Elizabeth Nolan Brown, "'Pregnant? Don't Want To Be?' Ads at South Dakota Gas Stations Spark First Amendment Battle," Reason, January 12, 2026. https://reason.com/2026/01/12/pregnant-dont-want-to-be-ads-at-south-dakota-gas-stations-spark-first-amendment-battle// .

101 NewsCenter1 Staff, "South Dakota, Mayday Health reach abortion pill ad settlement," News Center 1, March 9, 2026. https://www.newscenter1.tv/south-dakota-mayday-health-reach-abortion-pill-ad-settlement

102 *As Good as It Gets*, directed by James L. Brooks, (Sony Pictures Entertainment, 1997).

103 Gary M. Atkinson, "The Morality of Abortion," *International Philosophical Quarterly*, 14.2 (September 1974): 362.

104 David Boonin, *A Defense of Abortion* (Cambridge, NY: Cambridge University Press, 2003), xiv.

105 Planned Parenthood used to use the word "baby" in discussing abortion. In their pamphlet, "Plan Your Children for Health and Happiness," *Planned Parenthood Federation of America*, they note "An abortion kills the life of a baby after it has begun." Multiple versions of this pamphlet exist, but the wording among them is virtually identical. The one from which I quote here is an original in my possession. While it does have an address on the back for Planned Parenthood, it does not include a zip code. That would date this particular pamphlet before 1963, the date the zip code was mandated in the U.S. Photographs of this pamphlet can be found at https://speakerforlife.com/resources/.

106 Mary Elizabeth Williams, "So what if abortion ends life?" *Salon*, January 23, 2013, https://www.salon.com/test/2013/01/23/so_what_if_abortion_ends_life/

107 Warren M. Hern and Billie Corrigan, "What About Us? Staff Reactions to D & E," *Advances in Planned Parenthood*, 15:1, Excerpta Medica, 1980. Originally presented at the Association of Planned Parenthood Physicians in San Diego, October 26, 1978. https://www.drhern.com/wp-content/uploads/2018/05/staff-reaction-de.pdf.

108 Ibid. 5.

109 Ibid. 4-5.

110 Kimberly Ells, *The Invincible Family*, (Washington, D.C.: Regnery Gateway, 2020), 1.

111 Caroline Kitchener, "Alone in a bathroom" *Washington Post*, April 11, 2024

112 "White Dudes for Harris" unedited campaign call: https://www.youtube.com/watch?v=dnnKXuYcDU0, July 29, 2024. Buttigeig remarks: 19:22 – 24:15.

113 Christopher Kaczor, " *The National Catholic Bioethics Quarterly*, 5.2 (Summer 2005): 301. https://digitalcommons.lmu.edu/cgi/viewcontent.cgi?article=1109&context=phil_fac.

114 Rosalind Moran and Leslie Zhao, "Artificial Wombs Will Change Abortion Rights Forever," *Wired*, April 3, 2023. https://www.wired.com/story/ectogenesis-reproductive-health-abortion/. See also Elizabeth Chloe Romanis, "Abortion & 'artificial wombs': would 'artificial womb' technology legally empower non-gestating genetic progenitors to participate in decisions about *how* to terminate pregnancy in England and Wales?,"*Journal of Law and the Biosciences*, 8:1 (January-June 2021) https://academic.oup.com/jlb/article/8/1/lsab011/6279500. Romanis asserts that the mother's right not to become a parent outweighs the father's right to become a parent. The argument asserts, but does not prove, that the mother and father are not already parents of a living child.

115 Alberto Giubilini and Francesca Minerva, "After-Birth Abortion: Why Should the Baby Live?" *Journal of Medical Ethics*, 39 (2013): 263.

116 "Abortion Stigma," *Planned Parenthood Advocacy Fund of Massachusetts, Inc.* https://www.plannedparenthoodaction.org/planned-parenthood-advocacy-fund-massachusetts-inc/abortion-stigma.

117 Testimony of Dr. Colleen McNicholas, Chief Medical Officer Planned Parenthood of the St. Louis Region and Southwest Missouri, United States Senate Committee on the Judiciary "A Post-*Roe* America: The Legal Consequences of the *Dobbs* Decision" July 12, 2022. https://www.judiciary.senate.gov/imo/media/doc/Testimony%20-%20McNicholas%20-%202022-07-12.pdf

The live version of McNicholas' comments differs slightly from the published statement. You can see her testimony here: https://www.youtube.com/watch?v=72066J12kPE beginning at 44:12 and ending at 49:13.

118 Deidre McPhillips, "Under strict abortion law, Texas had nearly 10,000 more births than expected in the last nine months of 2022, research suggests," *CNN*, July 6, 2023. https://www.cnn.com/2023/07/06/health/texas-abortion-law-births/index.html?amp=&amp=&amp=.

119 Auger N, Brousseau É, Ayoub A, Fraser WD., "Second-trimester abortion and risk of live birth." *American Journal of Obstetrics and Gynecology*. 2024 Jun;230(6):679.e1-679.e9. doi: 10.1016/j.ajog.2023.11.004. Epub 2023 Nov 7. PMID: 37939985. Also located here: https://www.sciencedirect.com/science/article/abs/pii/S0002937823008062

120 Ibid.

121 "Abortion Care," *The American College of Obstetricians and Gynecologists*, https://www.acog.org/womens-health/faqs/induced-abortion.

122 "Fact Sheet: Pregnancy," *National Institute of Child Health and Human Development*, https://www.nichd.nih.gov/health/topics/factsheets/pregnancy.

123 "Twenty-One States Announce Historic Governor-Led Reproductive Freedom Alliance" https://www.gov.ca.gov/2023/02/21/twenty-states-announce-historic-governor-led-reproductive-freedom-alliance/

124 "About the Alliance," *Reproductive Freedom Alliance,* 2026. https://reprofreedomalliance.org/about-us/.

125 "Reproductive Justice," *In Our Own Voice: National Black Women's Reproductive Justice Agenda,* 2026. https://blackrj.org/our-causes/reproductive-justice/.

126 Unfortunately, the wall protecting elderly, infirm, or depressed post-born human beings from those who would intentionally kill them is breaking down. See Canada's MAID program or the rise of euthanasia in Europe.

127 The Cornyn/Bridges exchange can be found here: https://www.youtube.com/watch?v=72066I12kPE beginning at 1:58:00 and ending at 1:59:47. It begins with a discussion of systemic racism, but moves quickly into the exchange noted.

128 Chesterton wrote in *What's Wrong With the World* in 1910: "The Christian ideal has not been tried and found wanting. It has been found difficult; and left untried."

129 Harry Blamires, *A Defence of Dogmatism*, London: S.P.C.K, 1965, 6-7.

130 Ron E. Hassner, "From Which River to Which Sea? College students don't know, yet they agree with the slogan," *Wall Street Journal*, December 5, 2023. https://www.wsj.com/articles/from-which-river-to-which-sea-anti-israel-protests-college-student-ignorance-a682463b?mod=opinion_lead_pos11.

131 Ibid.

132 Ibid.

133 Adam Beam, "California may end travel ban to states with anti-LGBTQ laws," *AP News*, March 29, 2023. https://apnews.com/article/california-travel-ban-republican-states-lgbt-discrimination-d173fbf507db2c019eb336a828dd262a.

134 James Freeman, "Will California Law Allow UCLA to Play in the Big Ten?" *Wall Street Journal*, July 8, 2022. https://www.wsj.com/opinion/will-california-law-allow-ucla-to-play-in-the-big-ten-11657315232?mod=article_inline.

135 James Freeman, "UCLA's Big Ten Story," *Wall Street Journal*, July 19, 2022. https://www.wsj.com/articles/uclas-big-ten-story-11658269450?mod=opinion_lead_pos11.

136 Nicholas Goldberg, "Forget California's travel ban on anti-LGBTQ states. Engage instead," *Los Angeles Times*, April 17, 2023. https://www.latimes.com/opinion/story/2023-04-17/california-travel-ban-boycott-states-lgbtq-toni-atkins.

137 Ibid.

138 Full text of the bill can be found here: https://legiscan.com/CA/text/SB447/2023

139 Ibid.

140 "Procedural Abortion," *Planned Parenthood of Illinois*, 2026. https://www.plannedparenthood.org/planned-parenthood-illinois/patient-resources/abortion-services/procedural-abortion.

141 Katha Pollitt, *Pro*, (New York: Picador, 2014), 69.

142 Senator Dick Durbin, "The Assault on Reproductive Rights in a Post-*Dobbs* America," United States Senate, Committee on the Judiciary, April 26, 2023. https://www.congress.gov/event/118th-congress/senate-event/LC73533/text

143 Keith L. Moore, Mark G. Torchia and T.V.N Persaud, *The Developing Human: Clinically Oriented Embryology*, (Philadelphia, PA: Elsevier, 2020), 11.

144 Dr. Jerome Lejeune, professor of fundamental genetics at the University of Rene Descartes, who discovered the genetic basis for Down's Syndrome, testifying before the Subcommittee on the Separation of Powers of the U.S. Senate Committee on the Judiciary – April 23, 1981.

"At two months of age, the human being is less than one thumb's length from the head to the rump. He would fit with ease into a nutshell, but everything is there: hands, feet, head, organs, brain, all are in place. His heart has been beating for a month already. Looking closely you would see the palm creases... with a good magnifier the fingerprints could be detected. Every document is available for a national identity card...The human nature of the being from conception to old age is not a metaphysical contention; it is plain evidence."

145 "A New Ethic for Medicine and Society," *California Medicine: The Western Journal of Medicine*, (September 1970) 68.

146 "The Gift of Life," *Health Education Service*, N.Y. State Department of Health, 1951. For photo images of this booklet, including the back stamp showing it was distributed by Planned Parenthood Federation of America, please visit https://speakerforlife.com/resources/

147 C.S. Lewis, *The Abolition of Man*. (New York: MacMillan, 1947), 16-17.

148 "Amaze" *Influence Watch*, https://www.influencewatch.org/organization/amaze/.

149 ideaMachine Studio, "Amaze Video 1 – Our Bodies," *YouTube*. https://www.youtube.com/watch?v=w6ZEqYS6kbU.

150 Miriam@ Planned Parenthood, "I want to transition. How old do you have to be to get hormone therapy?" *Planned Parenthood*, October 13, 2025. https://www.plannedparenthood.org/blog/i-want-to-transition-how-old-do-you-have-to-be-to-get-hrt.

151 "2019: The World's Most Innovative Companies – Honorees by Sector," Fast Company, 2019. https://www.fastcompany.com/most-innovative-companies/2019/sectors/education.

152 "California Abortion Access" State of California, 2025. https://www.cdph.ca.gov/programs/ohe/abortion/pages/home.aspx.

153 Rahul Pandita, "Baby Doll Market Size and Share Forecast Outlook 2025 to 2035," *Future Market Insights*, September 15, 2025. https://www.futuremarketinsights.com/reports/baby-doll-market.

154 Ibid.

155 "A Never Before Seen Look At Human Life In The Womb | Baby Olivia," *Live Action*, YouTube, August 9, 2021. https://www.youtube.com/watch?v=S-lQOooYAs8. If YouTube removes this video, you can access it directly through the Live Action website here: https://babyolivia.liveaction.org/index.html. There is also a "Baby Oliver" video.

156 The board book can be acquired here: https://shop.liveaction.org/products/baby-olivia-board-book

157 Education Resource Fund, https://erf.science/#children-science-documentaries,

158 John Ensor, "Tiny Missionaries," *PassionLife PHO Worldwide*, Newsletter, June 23, 2026

159 Education Resource Fund, https://erf.science/.

160 Genesis 1:26

161 Genesis 1:28

162 Psalm 139:14

163 Exodus 20:13

164 Proverbs 24:11-12

165 Jeremiah 32:35

166 Luke 18:15-17; Mark 10:13-16

167 "Plan Your Children for Health and Happiness," *Planned Parenthood Federation of America*, no date. There are multiple versions of this pamphlet, but the wording between them is virtually identical. The one from which I quote here is an original in my possession. While it does have an address on the back for Planned Parenthood, it does not include a zip code. That would date this particular pamphlet before 1963, the date the zip code was mandated in the U.S. Photographs of this pamphlet can be found at https://speakerforlife.com/resources/.

168 Stephen D. Schwarz, *The Moral Question of Abortion* (Chicago, IL: Loyola University Press, 1990), 15-16.

169 Christopher Kaczor, *The Ethics of Abortion: Women's Rights, Human Life, and the Question of Justice* (New York, NY: Routledge, 2011) 143.

170 "Abortion Procedures," *Abort73.com*, https://abort73.com/abortion/abortion_techniques/ and "Abortion Pictures" https://abort73.com/abortion/abortion_pictures/.

171 Abortion No, https://abortionno.org/, 2026.

172 I discuss this in great detail in *Contenders*, 163-164.

173 Lyman Stone, "Promise and Peril: The History of American Religiosity and Its Recent Decline," *American Enterprise Institute*, April 30, 2020. https://www.aei.org/research-products/report/promise-and-peril-the-history-of-american-religiosity-and-its-recent-decline/.

174 Tracy F. Munsil, "New Research Shows Even Committed Christians Struggle with Application, As Overwhelming Majority of U.S. Adults Lack Biblical Basics," *2026 American Worldview Inventory – Report #2*, March 24, 2026. https://web.arizonachristian.edu/CRC/2026/AWVI-2026_Report_2-BWV_Eight_Categories.pdf.

175 Luisa Blanchfield, "Abortion and Family Planning-Related Provisions in U.S. Foreign Assistance Law and Policy," *Congress.gov*, July 15, 2022. https://www.congress.gov/crs-product/R41360.

176 "Tennessee Prostitution Laws" *Decriminalize Sex Work*, 2026. https://decriminalizesex.work/tennessee-prostitution-laws/.

177 Cassandra Webb, "New law prohibits organizations that offer abortions from teaching sex education in Arkansas schools," *KARK.com*, April 26, 2021. https://www.kark.com/news/local-news/new-law-prohibits-organizations-that-offer-abortions-from-teaching-sex-education-in-arkansas-schools/.

178 Rebecca Klapper, "Iowa Supreme Court Allows State to Ban Planned Parenthood From Conducting Sex Ed Classes," *Newsweek*, June 30, 2022. https://www.newsweek.com/iowa-supreme-court-allows-state-ban-planned-parenthood-conducting-sex-ed-classes-1605725.

179 Rolanda Donelson, "Texas Governor Signs Bill to Stop the Mailing of Medication Abortion to Texans," *KFF*, September 22, 2025. https://www.kff.org/quick-insights/texas-governor-signs-bill-to-stop-the-mailing-of-medication-abortion-to-texans/.

180 Enrolled House Bill No. 1168. https://www.oklegislature.gov/cf_pdf/2025-26%20ENR/hB/HB1168%20ENR.PDF.

181 For a current list of cities and counties with Sanctuary Cities for the Unborn ordinances, see https://sanctuarycitiesfortheunborn.org/incorporated-cities and https://sanctuarycitiesfortheunborn.org/counties

182 "Comanche County SCFTU Guidesheet," *Sanctuary Cities for the Unborn*, May 26, 2026.

183 The Comstock Act, though still a part of federal law, has not been enforced, and a number of Supreme Court decisions have weakened it.

184 "Need an Abortion and Need Help?" *Planned Parenthood of Tennessee and North Mississippi*, 2026. https://www.plannedparenthood.org/planned-parenthood-tennessee-and-north-mississippi/patient-navigation.

185 "Abortion assistance: Kroger to offer up to $4,000 of out-of-state travel costs for employees seeking abortion" *WCPO Cincinnati*, https://www.wcpo.com/news/local-news/hamilton-county/cincinnati/abortion-assistance-kroger-to-offer-up-to-4-000-of-out-of-state-travel-costs-for-employees-seeking-abortion.

186 Tess Bonn, "Here Are the Major U.S. Companies Covering Abortion Travel Costs," *Katie Kouric Media*, August 21, 2022. https://katiecouric.com/news/major-u-s-companies-covering-abortion-travel-costs/.

187 John Villasenor, writing in an otherwise pro-abortion leaning essay, still notes: "On balance, Supreme Court precedents regarding freedom of expression indicate that the provision of information (and advertising accompanied by information) about abortion should be protected under the First Amendment. But given that *Dobbs* itself upended precedent, it is difficult to predict how the Supreme Court might rule on future cases involving state attempts to limit speech about abortion." "Can a state block access to online information about abortion services?" *Brookings*, July 27, 2022. https://www.brookings.edu/articles/can-a-state-block-access-to-online-information-about-abortion-services/.

188 Senate Bill 276, 2024. https://www.legis.la.gov/legis/ViewDocument.aspx?d=1378429.

189 Rolley Haggard, "Incrementalism vs Immediatism in a Nutshell," *Free the States*, January 17, 2022. https://freethestates.org/2022/01/incrementalism-versus-immediatism-in-a-nutshell/.

190 The Cunningham vs. T. Russel Hunter debate is a video and probably one of the more comprehensive responses you are likely to see: https://www.youtube.com/watch?v=5oi4vVTae30&t=12s. The Klusendorf debate is audio only, and from 2024: https://ironsharpensironradio.com/2024/02/22/february-21-2024-show-with-jason-storms-and-scott-klusendorf-debating-abolition-vs-incrementalism-which-is-the-wisest-approach-for-christians-seeking-to-end-

the-slaughter-of-infants-through-abort/. Craig Ireland, "Clean Hands, Dead Children," *Craig's Substack*, June 7, 2026. https://craigireland.substack.com/p/clean-hands-dead-children. Scott Klusendorf, *The Case for Life*, (Wheaton, IL: Crossway, 2023), 331-338.

191 Mark Harrington, email interview, June 6, 2026.

192 Lincoln Brandenberg, email interview, June 12, 2026.

193 "A New Ethic for Medicine and Society," *California Medicine: The Western Journal of Medicine* (September 1970): 68.

194 T. Russell Hunter, "Does the Pro-Life Movement Hate Justice," *Abolitionists Rising*, April 9, 2026. Around minute 39 but also reflected in the title of the address. https://www.youtube.com/watch?v=LKSCnG5s3SI.

195 Emily MacFarland Miller, "Survey reveals public's skepticism about pastors," *The Christian Century*, March 1, 2017. https://www.christiancentury.org/news/survey-reveals-public-s-skepticism-about-pastors.

196 "Pastors Face Communication Challenges in a Divided Culture," *The Barna Group*, January 29, 2019. https://www.barna.com/research/pastors-speaking-out/.

197 "The Tricky Mix of Politics & Pastoring," *The Barna Group*, November 12, 2024. https://www.barna.com/trends/politics-pastoring/.

198 Lisa Cannon Green, "Women Distrust Church on Abortion," *Lifeway Research*, November 23, 2015. https://research.lifeway.com/2015/11/23/women-distrust-church-on-abortion/.

199 Alexander Bolton, "Hawley introduces bill to remove FDA approval for Mifepristone," *The Hill*, March 11, 2026. https://thehill.com/homenews/senate/5779756-hawley-fda-approval-mifepristone/.

200 Daniel Grossman, "New Data on Ulipristal Acetate and Misoprostol for Medication Abortion — A Step Forward? New England Journal of Medicine, January 23, 2025. https://evidence.nejm.org/doi/full/10.1056/EVIDe2400460.

201 See "What you should know about miscarriage signs, early miscarriage and more," *UC Davis Health*, July 17, 2024. https://health.ucdavis.edu/blog/cultivating-health/what-you-should-know-about-miscarriage-signs-causes-and-more/2024/07, and Stephanie Langmaid, "Miscarriage," *WebMD*, December 28, 2023. https://www.webmd.com/baby/pregnancy-miscarriage.

202 "Can a Doctor Tell You Took Abortion Pills? Mifepristone & Misoprostol Detection Explained," *Roxy Clinic*, April 19, 2026. https://roxyclinic.com/en/blog/can-providers-detect-abortion-pills.

203 Ibid.

204 Pawall Szpot, et. al. ""Determination of Mifepristone (RU-486) and Its Metabolites in Maternal Blood Sample after Pharmacological Abortion," *Molecules*, November 6, 2022, https://pmc.ncbi.nlm.nih.gov/articles/PMC9657224/.

205 You Zu, et. al. "Determination of misoprostol acid in human plasma by liquid chromatography coupled to tandem mass spectrometry," *Journal of Chromatography B*, June 1, 2007. https://www.sciencedirect.com/science/article/abs/pii/S1570023207000189.

206 Pawell Szpot, Olga Wachelko, and Marcin Zawadski, "Forensic Toxicological Aspects of Misoprostol Use in Pharmacological Abortions," *Molecules*, October 2022. https://www.researchgate.net/publication/364112807_Forensic_Toxicological_Aspects_of_Misoprostol_Use_in_Pharmacological_Abortions.

207 "Misoprostol Detection in Blood" *Gynuity Health Projects*, 2014. https://gynuity.org/assets/resources/factsht_misoinblood_en.pdf.

208 Sandra Poudrier, former co-founder and operations manager at RosVivo Therapeutics and former lab manager in the School of Medicine at University of Nevada, Reno, confirmed the expense of this instrumentation and methodology via email on May 26, 2026.

209 Szpot, "Forensic Toxicological Aspects of Misoprostol Use in Pharmacological Abortions"

210 Teresa Cisneros Burton, "New California Shield Law Protects Abortion Pill Patients, Prescribers and Pharmacists," *Ms.*, October 25, 2025. https://msmagazine.com/2025/10/25/california-shield-law-abortion-pill-names/.

211 "Powerful Reproductive Freedom Coalition Plays Key Role In Victory, Shows Momentum For Abortion Rights Win In November," *ACLU Ohio*, August 9, 2023. https://www.acluohio.org/press-releases/powerful-reproductive-freedom-coalition-plays-key-role-victory-shows-momentum/

212 Jo Ingles, "Ohio voters will decide a constitutional amendment on abortion. Here's what you need to know," *Statehouse News Bureau*, October 17, 2023. https://www.statenews.org/government-politics/2023-10-17/ohio-voters-will-decide-a-constitutional-amendment-on-abortion-heres-what-you-need-to-know

213 Andryanna Sheppard, "Question 6 asks voters if abortions should be legal in Nevada," *Fox 5 Las Vegas*, November 1, 2024. https://www.fox5vegas.com/2024/11/01/question-6-asks-voters-if-abortions-should-be-legal-nevada/

214 Many hormonal "contraceptives" also act as abortifacients, representing another area where increased education is necessary.

215 "Abortion Surveillance Findings and Reports," *Centers for Disease Control*, November 27, 2024. https://www.cdc.gov/reproductive-health/data-statistics/abortion-surveillance-findings-reports.html.

216 Elaine Godfrey, "Warren Hern: The Abortion Absolutist," *The Atlantic,* May 12, 2023. https://www.theatlantic.com/politics/archive/2023/05/dr-warren-hern-abortion-post-roe/674000/.

217 1 Kings 19:10.

218 J. Budziszewski, "Open Our Eyes," *Touchstone*, March/April 2026, 18-19.

219 Kim Hayes, "Mariah's Story: Beauty From Ashes." *Pregnancy Help News*, September 2, 2021. https://pregnancyhelpnews.com/mariah-s-story-beauty-from-ashes.

220 Mariah, "'For the First Time in My Life, I Started to Feel True Support': My Experience at a Pregnancy Resource Center," *Daily Signal*, October 17, 2022. https://www.dailysignal.com/2022/10/17/staffers-pregnancy-resource-center-were-my-life-preservers/.

221 Ibid.

222 Hayes, "Mariah's Story."

223 "Her Story," *Bakersfield Pregnancy Center*, March 21, 2023. https://www.youtube.com/watch?v=bFJOsDqMw8g.

224 Erin Rogers, personal email, June 4, 2026.

225 Budziszewski, "Open Our Eyes," 19.

226 "Total number of abortion providers in the United States from 1982 to 2020, by facility type," *Statista*, January 2023, https://www.statista.com/statistics/1400884/number-of-abortions-providers-by-facility-type-in-the-us/.

227 "Abortion in the United States," *Guttmacher*, March 2026. https://www.guttmacher.org/fact-sheet/induced-abortion-united-states.

228 "What is a Pregnancy Center?" *Heartbeat International*, 2026. https://www.heartbeatinternational.org/our-work/what-is-a-pregnancy-center.

229 "Postal Facts" *USPS*, 2025. https://facts.usps.com/delivery-points/.

230 Adam Scheidler (@Scheidsa). "This may be the song of the summer," *X*, May 14, 2026. https://x.com/Scheidsa/status/2055055545992626397.

231 Charles Curran (@charliebcurran), "LA is worth saving. Vote Spencer Pratt," *X*, May 5, 2026. https://x.com/charliebcurran.

232 Neil Postman, *Amusing Ourselves to Death*, (NY:Penguin Books, 1985), 99-100.

233 "She now sees abortion as a human rights injustice!" Protect Life Michigan, May 21, 2026. https://www.youtube.com/watch?v=BwGE4J8QoPo.

234 Michael Sherrard, phone interview by author, June 3, 2026.

235 You can still view all of the videos at Apologetics Inc.'s website: https://apologetics.org/prolife/.

236 Trevor Polo, "Operation Zero: 2024 Impact Report," PDF. 2024.

237 For more information, go to https//makeabortionhistory.org.

238 Mark Harrington, "Make Abortion History Summer 2025 Impact Report." PDF. 2026.

239 I was first introduced to this concept in Tolkien's essay "On Fairy Stories" which can be hard to find in print. You can read the essay here: https://coolcalvary.com/wp-content/uploads/2018/10/on-fairy-stories1.pdf.

240 Phil. 4:15-20.

241 "Zebrafish Embryo Growing Its Elaborate Sensory Nervous System | 2018 Nikon Small World," *Nikon Microscope Solutions*, September 27, 2018. https://www.youtube.com/watch?app=desktop&v=lQLsyf64xak.

242 Kirk Walden, *The Wall* (Nashville, TN: LifeTrends, 2013), 77.

243 "California Abortion Access," *California Department of Public Health*, 2025. https://www.cdph.ca.gov/Programs/OHE/abortion/Pages/Home.aspx. California used to host a site like this at abortion.ca.gov which now points to the other site above in this note. I think the original URL may have been deemed too inflammatory.

244 "What California is doing to protect abortion access," *California Department of Public Health*, 2025. https://www.cdph.ca.gov/Programs/OHE/abortion/Pages/your-rights/state-action.aspx.

245 “SCV Pregnancy Center Press Conference,” May 25, 2023. https://www.youtube.com/watch?v=uWhBvFUxZ30.

246 “Resources, Information, and Help for New and Expecting Mothers” https://moms.gov, 2026.

247 Texas Family Resources, https://www.familyresources.texas.gov.

248 AI, Summary of search results for “alliance pro-life governors,” June 3, 2026.

249 Kerstin Hering, “Life In Cuba,” *World*, May 2026, 84-89. https://wng.org/articles/life-in-cuba-1775233125.

About the Author

Dr. Marc Newman, president of Speaker for Life, galvanizes Christian leaders into advocates and champions for the preborn. Marc has trained thousands of speakers nationwide in communication skills. Through the Contend for Life conferences he teaches, he's equipped over a thousand pastors to better teach on life issues, along with thousands of laypeople to make the scientific, moral, and biblical case for life. Marc keynotes fundraising banquets each year that raise millions of dollars for pregnancy help centers and clinics.

Marc began his academic career as the Director of Speech and Debate at the University of California, Irvine, and he has served as a professor at both Palomar College and Regent University, teaching public speaking, debate, and the rhetoric of mass media. He's appeared on Fox News and in *Time* magazine. He's the author of *Contenders: A Church-Wide Strategy to Unmask Abortion, Defeat Its Advocates, Empower Christians, and Change the World.*

www.ingramcontent.com/pod-product-compliance
Lightning Source LLC
LaVergne TN
LVHW052257200926
848481LV00002B/392
* 9 7 8 1 7 3 5 1 9 6 2 4 4 *